SWEAT
SWEAR
SMILE

Lean Muscle for Life with Australia's Master Personal Trainer
FRED LIBERATORE

SWEAT
SWEAR
SMILE

FOREWORD BY MATT PRESTON
Food writer and TV & radio presenter

First published in 2021 by Dean Publishing
PO Box 119
Mt. Macedon, Victoria, 3441
Australia
deanpublishing.com

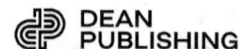

Copyright © Fred Liberatore

All rights reserved. No part of this publication may be reproduced, stored in a retrieval system or transmitted in any way or by any means, electronic, mechanical, photocopying, recording or otherwise, without the prior written permission of the publisher.

Cataloguing-in-Publication Data
National Library of Australia
Title: Sweat Swear Smile — Lean Muscle for Life with Australia's Master Personal Trainer
Edition: 1st edn
ISBN: 978-1-925452-31-0
Category: Health/Fitness/Nutrition

The views and opinions expressed in this book are those of the author and do not necessarily reflect the official policy or position of any other agency, publisher, organization, employer or company. Assumptions made in the analysis are not reflective of the position of any entity other than the author(s) — and, these views are always subject to change, revision, and rethinking at any time.

The author, publisher or organizations are not to be held responsible for misuse, reuse, recycled and cited and/or uncited copies of content within this book by others.

This book is not intended as a substitute for the medical advice of physicians. The reader should regularly consult a physician in matters relating to his/her health and particularly with respect to any symptoms that may require diagnosis or medical attention. The ideas within this book are only the opinion of the author and are not intended to replace any medical advice or diagnose health issues.

*This book is dedicated to you,
the inquisitive and brave reader that
has picked up this book in determination for a
better, fitter, stronger version of yourself.*

*It's dedicated to unlocking that part
of you that lives for no regrets,
that wants to find out what you're
truly capable of once and for all.*

*This book will show you the door
to a physically stronger life and
now you are here, I know you have the
courage to open it and step through.*

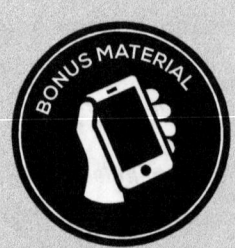

Fred is sharing bonus material.

In order to receive this,
simply email him at
info@leanmuscle.com.

CONTENTS

Foreword ix

Introduction: A Fitness Legacy xiii

Chapter 1: The Birth Of Realfit 1

Chapter 2: Mindset Is Everything 17

Chapter 3: Body 51

Chapter 4: Nutrition 71

Chapter 5: Exercises 91

Chapter 6: Workout 111

Chapter 7: Case Studies 129

Chapter 8: Work With Me 143

Chapter 9: Conclusion 159

Special Thanks To Some Very Special People 167

About The Author 173

Endnotes 175

Fred's Tips 181

FOREWORD
MATT PRESTON

Meet Fred Liberatore for the first time and you'll see he is a tightly coiled ball of energy like one of those hard rubber, high-bounce balls you used to play with as a kid. His enthusiasm almost overwhelms you. Here's a man whose whole life, whether as a wrestler, body-builder or trainer, has all been about peak fitness. For him that's his Everest, me I just want to make it up the stairs without puffing.

And it is this that makes Fred's approach to training so refreshing. He understands that one person's 50kg one-armed rows is another's 5kg farmer's walk (don't worry Fred will introduce you to the joys of both of these exercises soon enough!).

He realises that everyone has their own threshold and Fred takes pleasure in helping you beat each of these thresholds, no matter how small or how big, and no matter how they morph, as they will, as you become stronger and fitter following the advice in this book.

SWEAT

I met Fred Liberatore for the first time a little after I'd finished on *Masterchef* when I finally, after 11 years, had some time on my hands and could no longer justify prevaricating over getting back into training.

He came highly recommended by a mate who was willing to drive over two hours from his home in Benalla for Fred's tender mercies and the results that they offer. If Frank was willing to drive all that way then the 5 minutes from my house to Fred's gym was hardly a barrier.

The first thing you notice about Fred when you meet him is his energy – both mental and physical. He talks non-stop during sessions asking questions, sounding out how you are going, throwing out terrible jokes, and like all the very best trainers, he knows exactly how much harder he can push you. You'll find there's always a little bit more – until there isn't!

I've yet to come out of a session without having worked up a sweat: sometimes without even noticing it until I've come out to the car and my arms or legs no longer seemingly want to work anymore! It's a sort of delicious incapacity however that leaves you feeling so much stronger in the long run.

SWEAR

It took just 15 minutes of my second session with Fred before I swore at him. I was struggling through some chest reps after waaaay too long away from a gym, "12 more?! You sadistic bastard!" is, I think, what I said. There might have been a lot more expletives used than that...

Fred's reaction was just to laugh. He loved it. "It tells me I'm working you hard enough," he smirked.

OK, he probably just smiled but through my jaundiced eyes and a veil of perspiration it looked like a smirk.

So I'm very glad that "swear" has made it into the title of this his first book because if you are doing things right you should be swearing at Fred occasionally when following his advice for a better life. Whether he's advising you to give up coffee, eat more lean meats like his beloved kangaroo or spend an extra five minutes on the VersaClimber (don't ask, you don't want to know what this instrument of torture is but luckily for you it's too big to fit in this book!).

SMILE

I'm delighted to say however that the smiles should outweigh any of the challenges of training with Fred.

Over the time Fred's been training me that's the other great thing, the fact that he'll always make you smile. Perhaps not from his textbook lines of "Dad joke" humour or from his near obsession with sardines and sweet potato but just from the warmth and concern that he shows to everyone who comes into his gym to train.

There's no doubt if it wasn't fun training with Fred I would have given up a long time ago, found some excuse – work, lockdown, injury, interstate business, etc – and slowly slipped out of the frame. After all where's the joy of going to the gym if it's all pain? There has to be some form of enjoyment there and I hope that you find that in the pages that follow.

So now it's time to enjoy your own personal journey with Fred. It will be serious, it will be challenging if you want it to be – and can I recommend that you push yourself because that's where the most satisfaction lies, but it will also be a whole lot of fun.

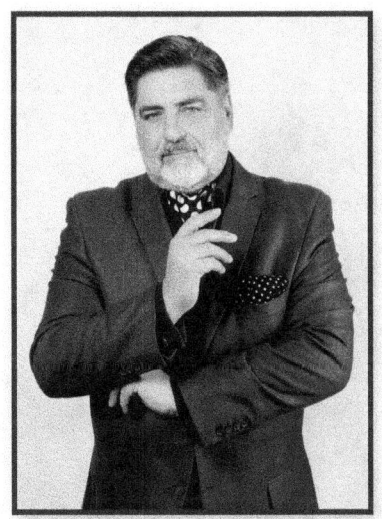

Even if there may be times when you do want to call Fred all the bad names under the sun – or you would if you had any breath left in your body!

Love you Freddie. You're my favourite brother too...

Matt Preston
Food writer and TV & radio presenter

INTRODUCTION

A FITNESS LEGACY

If this book inspires just one person to shake themselves out of the physical slump they find themselves in and propels them in a more positive and healthy direction, then I have achieved my goal.

These pages are more than a book for me; they are a fitness legacy that I feel so excited to share following my four fulfilling decades living and breathing this great industry from end to end.

I hope these words will empower ordinary people to find the motivation and strength that I know is within them. The duality of my personal and fitness journeys over so many years has resulted in incredible transformations not only for myself, but for my clients as well. This evolution continues each day that I live and work in the business that I love: helping people to find the best versions of their physical selves. This achievement has a wonderful impact on all aspects of their lives.

Imparting the lessons I've experienced over such a long time in this book is a small way to thank and give back to an industry that has been so inspirational and kind to me.

I am honoured to assist every individual who asks me to be a part of their fitness journey. As I watch them discover inner qualities they didn't know they possessed, I find myself learning something new from them, their challenges and how they dig deep to find the strength to overcome them. This experience with each person helps me to become a better version of myself too. What an amazing connection to look forward to each day!

I have been asked time and again to share my insights, my story, my experience — even my secrets — and through this book writing process, I have been able to reflect on the long and windy road that led to my health and fitness dreams coming true. This has added to my own personal growth in a whole new way.

Every client I work with knows they will receive more than just personal training. It's not simply physical training, we also train the mind to go beyond its former limitations. I have high expectations for my clients to succeed and this spurs each person on to make a commitment with me and with themselves and they work even harder than they thought possible. They know if they want results — real, tangible, life-changing results — then I am the guy for them.

FIRST...BACK TO THE '80s

What a buzz it's been for me to look back on my upbringing and early life that paved the way for my fitness aspirations and launched me into such a fulfilling career. My Italian born parents embraced the Aussie culture when they immigrated here in 1956. I had a fun, loving, working class upbringing around the inner northern suburbs of Melbourne. If you ask me, the '80s era had genuine spunk, a tough spirit and a straightforward style that taught us patience and gratitude. You couldn't get everything you wanted instantly, nor could you simply google answers to your questions. Life was discovered through experience and trial and error.

I remember jumping into my dad's zippy little Datsun on hot summer days. The air conditioning was useless so I'd madly crank the handle of the window down while trying not to burn myself on the scorching vinyl seat or the seatbelt.

As kids, we never relied on our parents to take us anywhere to see friends; that would have been a rare privilege but there were no play centres or adventure playgrounds back then anyway. So I was lucky to be able to walk or ride my bike around the neighbourhood to hang out with mates. Our parents trusted us to be home by curfew and we stuck to it probably out of fear; we all knew if we were late, they'd quickly take away our neighbourhood privileges and keep us grounded at home for ages.

We relied on our imaginations for entertainment. When we weren't searching for spiders and other creepy crawlies in the dunny in our backyard, we'd take a few bats and balls to the small park near our house and spend hours replaying memorable sporting moments from our AFL or cricket heroes. There was no internet, no Google, and no mobile phones. Those were the days.

Do you remember how nearly every second street corner used to have a phone booth on it? I memorised as many landline phone numbers of my friends as I could so I didn't have to carry around my little phone book from home. Although, the phone booths often had a directory chained to the back wall (if it hadn't already been ripped out), it was pretty much the bible of communication back then.

It only cost around 15-20 cents to make a call. However long distance calls, especially to Italy, cost a fortune and so we would try to call when the international call rate was low — otherwise it was a horrible shock when the phone bill arrived and we had called at the wrong time! My parents were conscious and careful with every cent they worked hard for and how it was spent.

My strongest memories are of the freedom and time I spent with good friends, without the endless rush, rush, rush and distractions of today. How funny it is now to think that you had to drop off your camera film to the camera store and then try not to lose your processing slip during the weeks and weeks of waiting for the film to be developed — it felt like ages.

I'd buy a little photo album all ready for when the pictures came back and occasionally I'd buy double copies so I could share them with my mates. But there was no option but to wait patiently for their return. That was life in the '80s; no instant gratification from a digital photo that you can delete if you don't like it, or share it instantly with someone on the other side of the world!

Owning music was another lesson in patience back then. Countless times I sat by the radio waiting for my favourite song to come on, my finger would hover over the 'record' button on the cassette player and I'd slam it down as soon as I heard the familiar opening bars of the song I wanted. I hated it when the DJ talked over the start of the song; it really ruined the playback.

When you ran out of blank tapes, you could simply record over the old songs you didn't want anymore. Making a mix tape of your favourite songs (it could take months) was a real achievement back then and giving someone the mixed tape you'd made was a way to show someone you *liked* them back then ☺.

If you loved a song enough, you could save up $5-10 pocket money to buy a cassingle — a cassette tape that only had the song you wanted on Side A, and a different version or bonus song on Side B. The cassingle was a strange fad that didn't last that long but was so typical of the '80s. The first actual album I bought was Michael Jackson's *Off the Wall* on cassette tape. I'll never forget the lady in the shop telling me I had hair like Michael Jackson because I had an afro. He was my idol so I took it as a huge compliment.

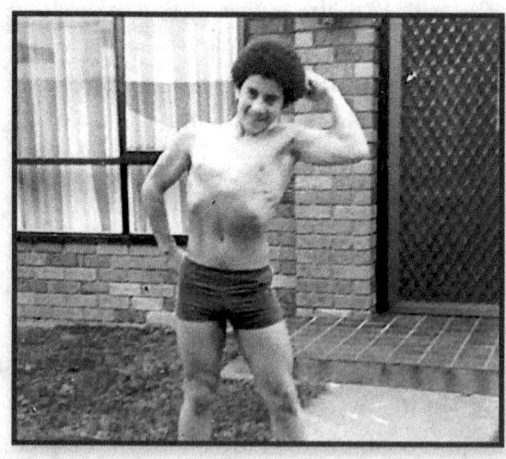

In summer, our parents would take my twin brother, Tony, and I down to the beach in Altona while our older siblings did their own thing. When we arrived, we would run and jump off the end of the pier, straight into the cool, welcoming shock of the salty water. There was no fear, just fun. Mum was a legend packing salami, sandwiches, olives and fresh bread. We would be ravenous by the time we ran up the sand for a break. We spent many family days like this together, a great memory I'll hold onto always.

Growing up with older siblings and a very competitive twin made me obsessed with exercise, health and nutrition. My brother Tony (aka Libba) ventured on to become one of the most famous footballers in VFL/AFL history.[1] Growing up, we would often be asked, "Who's older?" I would always shoot back, "Me, by ten minutes!" This was always a big deal to me; it was only ten minutes but I wanted people to know I was still the older brother. Maybe I thought it meant wiser too.

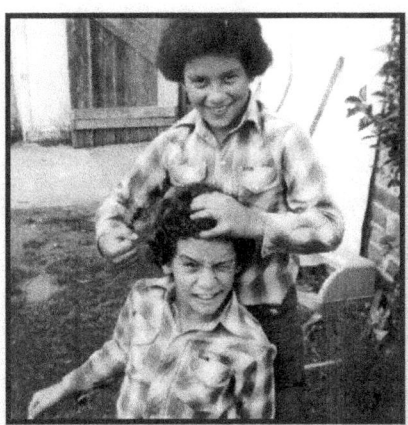
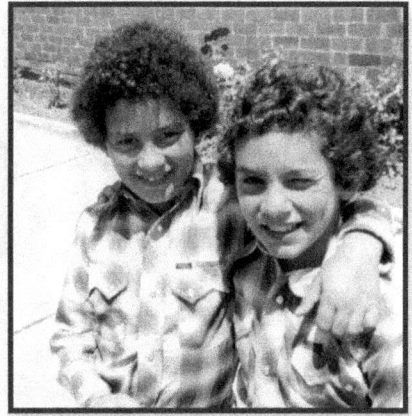

You'd think that twins would be born small, but Tony and I entered the world at a hefty 8.5 pounds (3.85 kg) each. It's hard to imagine my poor, tiny-framed mother Maria, holding 17 pounds. Well she did, and continues to remind us all the time! Mum has always been a devout practising Catholic and always reminded her children of the importance of having faith (she still does to this day). She would fire up the vacuum cleaner early on a Sunday morning as our wake-up call to get us to church on time.

Along with the value of faith, the importance of exercise was also driven deeply into our DNA. I think Mum also found it a great way to ensure we didn't destroy our family home; after all, boys will be boys. Mum embraced the Aussie fixation on sport and we played AFL football in the winter months and cricket during summer. It was not an option to stay home. We needed to choose a sport and run with it.

We would have to work hard to save enough money for those special footballs and cricket bats we wanted. We mowed lawns and did odd jobs for our neighbours until finally our goal was reached and we'd buy the latest equipment to improve our sporting prowess. We'd play in the nearby park for endless hours with our friends and cousins until it got too dark to see what we were doing and we'd scurry home as fast as we could, with sweaty smiles on our faces.

Each year, Tony and I would compete against each other in footy and often, either he or myself would win the Best and Fairest award for the season. I have to admit; footy gave me the foundation and groundwork to be the athlete I am today, especially playing at the senior level.

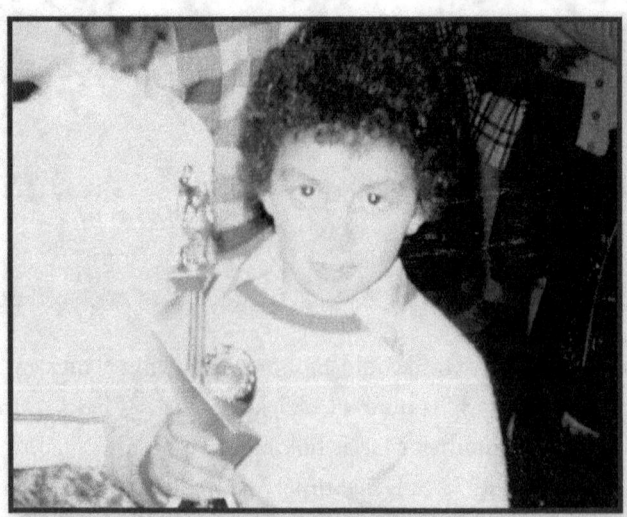

By employing a 'can do' attitude with grit and determination, both Tony and I tried out for the VFL Under-19 North Melbourne team. He was fast and very agile whereas I was slower and bulkier due to my thicker frame. My lower body muscle mass was starting to get in the way, especially during pre-season so speed and stamina was a challenge.

Around the age of 18, I found my passion for footy was dissolving and my drive to be more muscular was increasing. I realised football was not my calling or the path for me. After trying out with North Melbourne Under-19s the coach literally told me to get out after the first week. I was cut. I didn't blame him and we left on good terms. Such is the ruthlessness of elite sport.

Tony continued on and was very successful. As much as I enjoyed playing team sports, in all honesty, I was drawn to more solo sports where you can really test yourself individually. It was time to make some tough decisions with my footy career without procrastinating.

I wanted something different. I wanted to work my body from the inside-out. My frame started bulking up and at 19 years old, I already had well developed legs and was tipping the scales at 80+ kilograms and starting to see visible stretch marks a result of my increasing workouts. As a teen I saw stretch marks as a positive indicator that my muscles were expanding.

I was really getting into this fitness thing. I added wrestling to my list of sports, which by the way, I still find one of the most challenging sports out there. I joined the gym and continued to physically push myself further and further. Part of this drive came from the fact that I wanted to have my own identity, separate to the growing fame of my twin.

People began referring to me as Tony's twin brother. I didn't have a name to them; I was simply 'his brother'. I know they never meant any harm; it's how people relate to one another or how people make connections. Looking back now, I understand why I worked so hard to find something that was just mine, to carve out my own, very different identity to his.

Now don't get me wrong, I have always been incredibly proud of Tony and I still am. Tony found his passion much earlier than I did. There was never a feeling of being left out in my family; we were always loved and treated equally. I personally felt though, I needed to find out who I was, without being defined by what my very successful twin was achieving.

My parents taught me from a very young age the value of hard work and that nothing comes to you without commitment. I landed my first part-time work at a supermarket stocking shelves. I would then take my pay and re-invest in myself by subscribing to medical journals to educate myself on the human body, all the while working out daily to obtain the body I was envisioning in my mind.

I was fascinated by real case studies of people who had transformed their bodies by sculpting them to be muscular and healthy. It was an ideal I aspired to. So I decided to reinvent myself as an individual, to re-engineer my identity and find my own path in life. The more I read and researched about the fitness potential of the human body, the more I found myself absorbed by it. Bodybuilding was drawing me in more and more every day, and I liked that I only had one person to compete against: myself.

A MENTOR EMERGES

My older brother John witnessed my passion and appetite to learn more and decided to help me on my quest to be the athlete I was dreaming of.

The fitness industry in Australia began in the early '80s mainly marketed as aerobic exercise (who can forget the spandex wearing instructors on the TV show, *Aerobics OZ Style?*). While this may have been entertaining, there still wasn't much actual information out there about the science behind body and fitness. Quality gym equipment wasn't available either; it was clunky and poorly made at the best of times.

There was no easy way to improve muscle back then and we often had to improvise. One day John and I got creative with a few rusted, empty paint tins that were left over from when Dad painted the house. John saw their potential and made a barbell by filling them with cement and fixing an old rusty six-foot-long thick pipe between them.

I stumbled across a Spenby at my local Op shop. A Spenby was a chest expander with a quick-change snap link that would basically rip out any chest hair I had if I wasn't careful. I didn't care, I wanted it, and I refused to wait a minute longer. That Spenby didn't help me make friends, but the allure of John's homemade barbell brought friends from every direction.

The repetition of using the barbell to press, pull and squeeze, worked every imaginable muscle in my body. I worked out tirelessly in the bungalow behind our Brunswick home with only the streetlight from the laneway allowing me to see. After the workout I'd scoff down a dozen bananas and guzzle a carton of full cream milk for nutrients.

My somewhat athletic frame was adding real muscle and John could see I was taking this exercise stuff seriously. I felt proud of my new body. I would brag about a new stretch mark on my upper chest area and show off my body whenever I could. John bought me a membership to our local gym called Fitzys. I was stoked and overwhelmed at what John had done for me. It felt like all my Christmases had come at once.

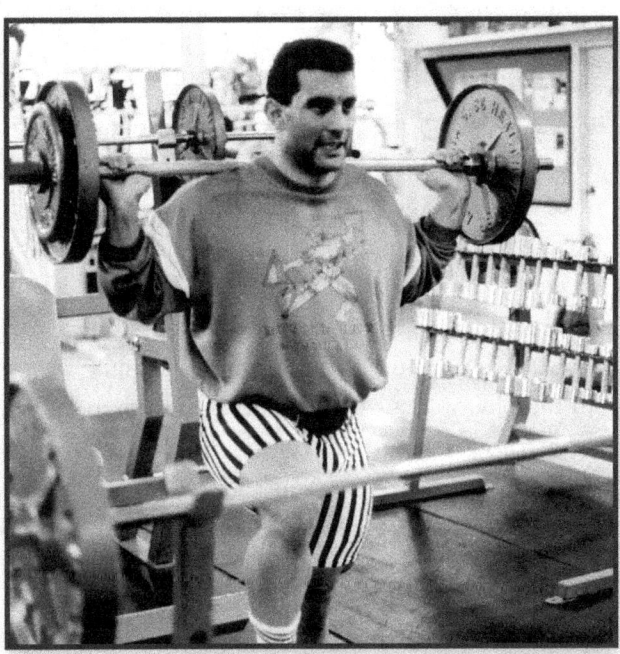

As soon as I stepped into that gym I was truly in muscle heaven. I saw bodybuilders with well-worn, ripped t-shirts, training their arses off, freely giving advice and spotting their fellow muscle builders with no mobile phone in sight. The good old days certainly were better without the devices. People would focus solely on what they were doing.

Not long after walking in the gym, I recognised a man from the magazines I subscribed to: a bodybuilder whom I worshipped. This guy literally had arms as big as my head. In my excitement, I ran over to him and blurted out, "Excuse me, how do I get big arms? What's a good exercise for a wide back? Can you show me how to do a skull crush?"

I was quickly told to back off and that if I wanted to see him, I would have to attend his seminar that evening. I was confused by his abrupt manner and the fact he was lying down with his feet elevated on a box reading a porno magazine!

At that moment, I realised I could become as built as he was with the right training and mindset. I could easily mirror his training style, not so much his reading style if you get my drift. My 'hero' did not end up meeting my expectations. He was egotistical and not a real advocate for health and wellbeing. He could have been using his time at the gym mentoring others. To me, this was a wasted opportunity. I believe every moment is a teachable moment and I knew straight away, that I never wanted to have the same attitude as him. I wanted to be a mentor, a coach and someone to inspire others to be better. Just as my brothers John and Tony were my mentors, guiding and encouraging me to be the best I could be.

As my interest continued, I could already boast a very impressive collection of fitness magazines that I had invested in from the newsagency. I would be constantly reading and learning about bodybuilders like Lee Haney, Arnold Schwarzenegger and Lou Ferrigno. I would carry a pocket-sized photo of my favourite bodybuilder in my wallet and had posters hanging behind my bedroom door.

Not only would I highlight the articles concerning my favourite athlete's diet and exercise programs, I would memorize them. That really heightened my interest in the science behind fat loss and the ultimate quest for lean muscle. I no longer went to the newsagency to read fitness magazines, instead I headed to the local library to delve deeper, sitting there for hours sifting through books on anatomy, learning how muscles worked and why.

I read research papers involving anything from the mindset behind weight loss and nutrition to exercise, fat loss and case studies around this. It would take me about a day to read through each article because I had to stop and check almost every word in the medical dictionary.

I had reached this point because I was over the smoke and mirror stuff you see in magazines promoting a miracle weight loss pill and potion. After years of reading about the 'latest and greatest' diet methods in magazines, I didn't know who or what to believe anymore. I found each magazine's newest diet method contradicted the diet method published in the previous month's edition. It was purely speculation; very few methods were based on science, while others were complete gibberish, defying the fundamental laws of thermodynamics and science.

When it came to losing weight and packing on lean muscle, every 'nutrition guru' and weight-loss personality had their own theory on what did and didn't work. Consumed by the hype, it was easy to ignore my previous doubts and think their absurd diet theory sounded logical (even though there was no scientific evidence to support the theories).

I noticed if an idea is published, and enough people accept it, it's perceived as true no matter whether it's accurate or not. I saw how magazines would recycle unproven diet programs and confuse the reader to drive up sales each month — it helped pioneer the instant gratification generation.

So that's how I became resolved to 'test and measure' everything and see what did and didn't work. This has become my personal fitness philosophy and I speak about it throughout the book. Through so many years of working with individuals of differing body types, different lifestyles, tastes and preferences, by testing and measuring various methods, I have developed a program to specifically focus on different areas of the body, and in conjunction with the best eating regime, my clients (and myself) are able to obtain the desired results in a realistic, sustainable timeframe.

Not long after this, around 1985, I started working at the council run gym at Broadmeadows Leisure Centre. When I wasn't working, I would wrestle. My obsession with fitness was at its peak and people were starting to notice.

My three goals when studying exercise, nutrition and mindset were to:
1. Learn everything I possibly could about nutrition and metabolism and its effects on the body.
2. Research those at the top of their game, break their model down and make it better.
3. Graduate with high marks as a gym instructor and massage therapist.

My obsession to learn about the human body led me to undergo a certificate in massage. Once qualified I offered sports massage from my parents' home to my fitness training partners who always complained about feeling sore. From massage I then studied and qualified as a Personal Trainer. Back when I graduated, personal training wasn't as big as it is now. You couldn't make a full time income out of it, so it began as a part time gig for me.

THE FITNESS INDUSTRY DOES NOT ALWAYS GET IT RIGHT

I understand that fitness companies want to advertise their businesses. But often their strategy involves propagating a feeling of guilt and physical inadequacy in society. Statements like:

Get your beach body now!
Fit into your bathing suit in 10 days!
Get a six-pack in 14 days!
Overindulged? Take this product!

These campaigns all imply you don't fit the idealised body. They also imply their superior product offers a magical 'quick fix' solution to your problem. Their focus is always on the extreme examples that are usually unattainable and target the masses, rather than focusing on the individual and creating sensible goals that apply to the person's unique situation.

Only the unscrupulous organisations hook clients in with enforced 12-month lock in contracts. Their business model is built on non-attendees and they will do anything to get them to sign on the dotted line. How does that make you feel? Like a faceless number? It's aggravating, isn't it?

On top of this, their websites show perfectly sculpted bodies. They propagate the message that looking good is the most important thing in life. The images that make up their publicity campaigns are smoke and mirrors, and represent a very small percentage of people who often make a living from their looks.

Those images are not realistic for most people. Even those few who do dedicate a lot of time to attend the gym, are still left feeling miserable and ignored when their gym does nothing to help them achieve their goals.

These companies do not cater for the real person balancing busy schedules trying to find time and genuine help for their own health. There are a range of 'normal' people that need slow, steady, solid and sustainable progress for their health. Loads of different body shapes fit into the 'normal' category and 'normal' is completely underrated in my experience.

In more recent times, I have seen positive shifts in the industry where workouts are becoming more functional. This means that even though some of these workouts seem repetitive and boring, their focus is on strengthening core muscles and the body as a whole. I also love that many places are now showing the practical value of transforming one's health through games, and I believe this should be the role of the fitness industry.

It sounds simple, but the joys of running, jumping and moving you felt as a child, can be found again by freeing up and strengthening those muscles. Fitness is fun so let's bring back playtime!

I encourage you to take everything you read or hear with a grain of salt and I invite you to test and measure to find out if it's true for you.

SWEAT SWEAR SMILE

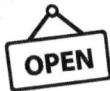

CHAPTER 1

THE BIRTH OF REALFIT

MY LIGHT BULB MOMENT

The world changed on September 11, 2001 when America's Twin Towers were attacked. The events of that day also triggered an epiphany for me to seize the day.

At the time, I was working in international freight forwarding. It was a good job, I travelled the world and the pay was good, but I knew it was not my true calling. As many do, I worked in order to pay bills and put food on the table. I was weight training in my spare time, fitness was still very important to me.

When the Towers were hit, my twin brother Tony was in New York on a football trip. He was also with Australian tennis champion Lleyton Hewitt celebrating his US Open victory against Pete Sampras. I didn't know it at the time, but Tony had left the Tower only 30 minutes before the attack and so thankfully he escaped before the devastation took place.

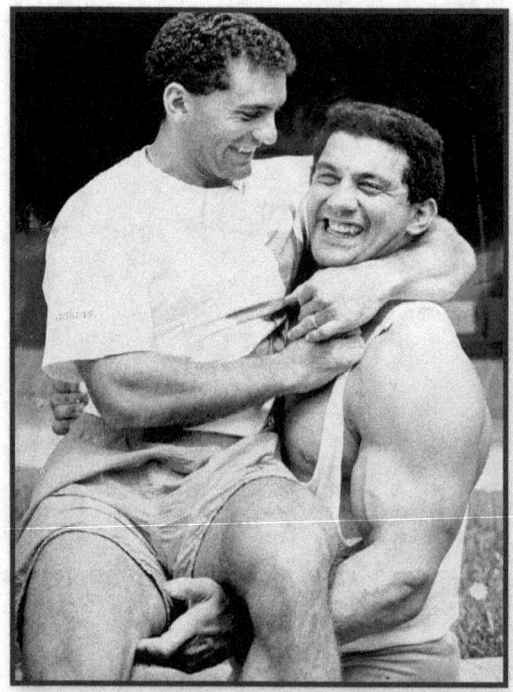

However, the waiting to find out if Tony was okay and not knowing what was happening struck me as a huge awakening. Everything became very clear suddenly, like a light bulb had finally shone the spotlight on my deepest passion.

At that moment, I knew I could not waste any more time doing something I didn't love. I walked straight into my boss's office and said, "Mike, I'm not living my best life. I've got to go," and I walked out, never looking back. I had the will to succeed and the passion for personal training so I chose to pursue my dream. It hasn't always been easy, but it has always been worth it.

I obtained a job in a gym and worked myself up the chain, making some fantastic connections. I would write up programs, put weights away, open up in the early hours of the morning and lock up late at night. I loved being involved and having great conversations with people about their health goals.

Throughout my four decades in fitness, I have worked in all facets of the industry. From amateur enthusiast, massage therapist, personal trainer for small and national gyms, competing and winning competitions, working with an Australian supplement company in brand development and running their challenges and also being known as Australia's 'Master Coach', I have done it all. As I began to win competitions, I had professional photos taken as a way to mark and remember my accomplishments.

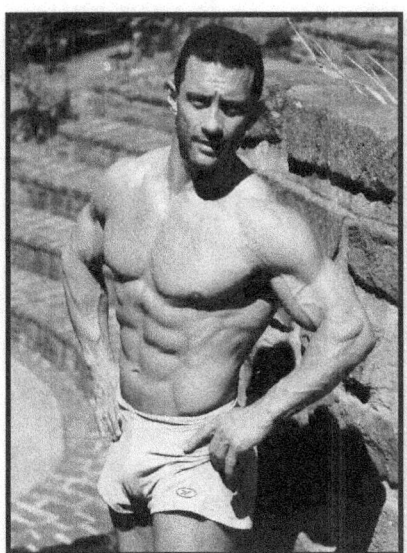
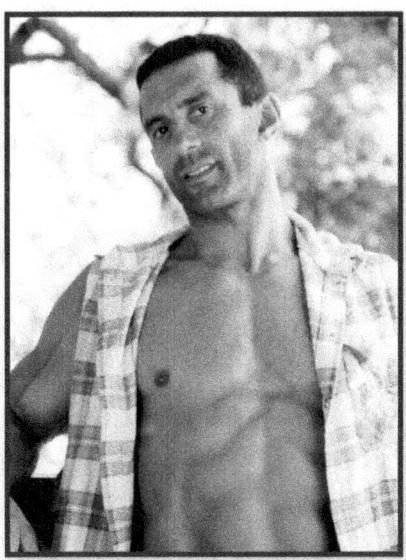

People would often look at me and say, "Wow Fred, I want your legs," or "How do you do it?" I developed such a depth of knowledge and breadth of experience that people were always coming up asking me for help. I would happily share any advice, I would write out a program for them if they asked, I'd write a list of what I was eating or give them tips on getting bigger legs.

My massage, anatomy and physiology background enabled me to give them information from a wider, more rounded perspective, often it wasn't just one thing that would help them move closer to their goal. It was about lifestyle changes too.

When I was training and saw someone doing an exercise wrong, it was really concerning because I know that incorrect technique can potentially be harmful. So I'd walk over and introduce myself and say, "Hey buddy, it looks like you're doing that exercise wrong and you could get hurt. Can I show you the right way to do it?" They were always happy to hear some advice and talk about their own journey.

FITNESS & FREEDOM

Finally my dream to open my own personal straining studio was taking shape; a place where I wasn't bound by the restraints of a large-scale franchise; a place of change and positivity, and where I had the freedom to really help and change people's lives.

I've always been genuinely passionate about helping clients close the gap in achieving their weight loss and/or optimal health goals with the bonus of incredible energy levels. I truly believe every 'body' is an athlete (most of us are just not Olympic athletes) and that everything starts from the ground up, your framework for moving forward.

I searched for a studio space for a very long time; it had to be the exact 'right' space that aligned with my philosophy and training style. I was excited to open Realfit Personal Training in Prahran (Victoria) in 2012 and later followed with a second smaller studio in nearby East Malvern in 2015.

I tried to make the two premises work for a few years, however, while I could replicate the system, I couldn't duplicate myself. I couldn't duplicate my knowledge and experience or be in two places at once, or nurture each member on their journey (people often came to the studio to connect with me). And so I ended up selling the Prahran studio in 2019.

After successfully establishing my bricks and mortar business I saw a need to reach people across all states of Australia as word got out that I was 'the' guy that could fix and transform people! I had already established the Lean Muscle brand back in the early '80s but never really did anything with it, and realised Lean Muscle could be a stand alone digital brand that compliments the RealFit brand and gave people an option to train with me in-person at RealFit or online with leanmuscle.com.

Now I am well into my 50s, and my passion for fitness, nutrition and health has not dissipated. It has only increased with time. I have since sold my facility and moved to the online world at leanmuscle.com, as well as now being a keynote speaker, travelling the world and delivering valuable content to companies. I have developed the ability to educate, inspire and make people laugh all at the same time!

The core of my business is still online transformations, whatever that looks like for each individual client – body changes, nutrition changes, reduced stress and anxiety, more confidence, better sleep, and so on. I am here to help facilitate the changes each client desires through a personalised training program, access to first-class training, no matter their location, and resources to support their journey.

I have kept to my promise of impacting individuals across all generations, making positive fitness and lifestyle changes. You can find my clients' success stories on my website leanmuscle.com.

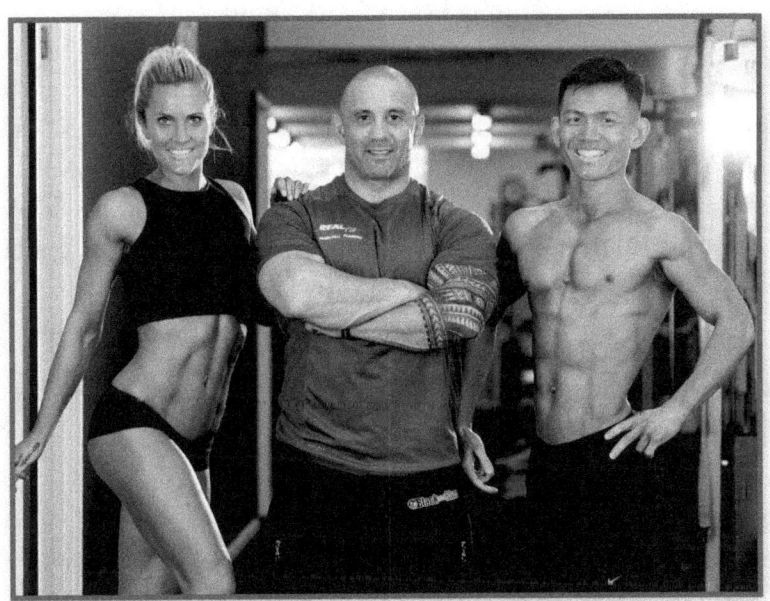

I am a lifelong student of strength and conditioning, consistently learning and improving my craft. The more I know, the more I can help you achieve your goals. I've invested in my growth with the below certifications and each certification covers the following:

- **Certified Level III & IV Personal Trainer** — functional training and injury management, nutritional guidance, anatomy, physiology and prescribing exercise, First Aid.
- **StrongFirst Kettlebell Level I & II Instructor** — kettlebell precision for developing, maximising, and maintaining strength.
- **Certified Health and Wellness Coach** — motivation, behaviour change (helping you overcome limiting beliefs), nutrition and weight management, holistic approaches to managing stress and increasing energy.
- **Massage Therapist** — functional anatomy and physiology, sports massage and therapeutic stretching.

If you've used a trainer in the past or currently use a trainer, do you know what their trainer certifications are? Most people don't ask, which astounds me! I encourage people to always ask a trainer what their qualifications are and whether they regularly update their professional development. This way you have an understanding of what they can (and can't) help you with.

WORKING WITH ALLIED HEALTH PROFESSIONALS

Most people will commence a journey of physical fitness after experiencing pain or a health scare. Supporting you is our purpose. Our focus is ensuring you achieve the goal you've set, helping you every step of the way as you navigate the physical work, mindset changes, nutrition and lifestyle changes to create and achieve your sustainable life moving forward.

I am fortunate that allied health professionals such as chiropractors, physiotherapists and other health professionals refer me to their clients. A personal trainer does work differently to a physiotherapist, yet in conjunction with them (and also initiating contact with their health professional if requested by the client) to achieve the best result for the client, especially if they are healing from an injury.

Do consult a recommended allied health professional so you can make an informed decision to achieve your goal. My colleagues in allied health understand how well we work together in supporting people's physical goals. Some recent testimonials:

> *"As a Chiropractor, I highly recommend Fred and the team at Realfit. Fred is a fantastic trainer and will get you incredible results. Awesome gym and awesome team!"*
>
> — **Jeremy from Centre 4 Health**

> *"Such a professional and amazing supportive environment! Thanks Fred and the Team. Can highly recommend."*
>
> — **Kate from The Chiro Tree**

MY FITNESS PHILOSOPHY

My philosophy has always been to show up and be present in every moment. I believe you must train smart, not just hard.

My personal formula is: Sweat — Swear — Smile.

I know I've had a great session if I've done all three of these. I don't take excuses. I think everyone needs to find something they love, stick to it and give it a real go, not just for a week but at least for a few months. You want to be able to build momentum and momentum tends to develop with training and commitment over time.

The beauty of sticking to something for a while is that you can always trump your last session. You can always reach for a new height or goal to outdo yourself. The only person you can truly compete against is yourself.

Every time I train, I grade myself and the session out of 10. I ask my clients to do the same. Think about how you are feeling at the beginning and throughout the session, and what could have been done better. Neither my clients nor I have ever been a 10. We usually hover around the 6-8 mark.

What I have experienced and witnessed is when you are consistent, your body and mind adapt and improve. My advice to you is to be present in the moment, have minimal distractions and be consistent. You may like to sit down with your diary and find some time you can dedicate to training and then lock it in!

I cannot emphasise enough that you really need to embrace nutrition, mindset and training when going down the fitness rabbit hole!

Let's look at my philosophy in more detail for a moment, as it is a core theme throughout the book.

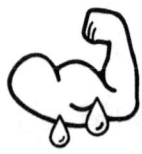

SWEAT

Sweat is the cooling mechanism for the body and proof you've pushed yourself in the workout. Much information can be researched that explains the significance of sweating. Sweating is a contributing factor to controlling body temperature, making sure that you do not overheat. The human mechanism is so intelligent, and innately understands what to do for its optimal function.

Additionally, sweating assists in dampening or moistening the palms, which helps with gripping. There are cases where some people may experience excessive sweating, which is known as hyperhidrosis. This condition has no known cause, but it can be managed by reducing excess body fat (I can help with that) and getting checked by your healthcare professional to make sure your hormones are in balance. Most people have normal sweating patterns in their lives caused by heat, working out and fever among other things.

Lack of sweat is an indication you are dehydrated. Hydrate throughout the day and before you commence your workout. One of the ways we can see how effectively we have worked out, is by the amount we have sweated. If you are working out, fully hydrated, and yet find you are not sweating (or sweating sufficiently), then you are not working out hard enough!

You must raise your heart rate enough to bring on a sweat and that is when you know you are working out to your personal limit, which can always be outdone in your next workout. Once the same routine no longer breaks you out in a sweat, it's time to up your game.

A lot gets said about the amount of sweat people produce. Some men think they are fitter than their female partners because they sweat more. But there is a simple explanation for this: while females may have more glands, male sweat glands produce more sweat.

Researchers found that females sweat less than males but still are able to maintain a normal body temperature. This is because females are more efficient sweaters than males. And why is this? Because female bodies evaporate sweat on their skin more efficiently, which cools down the body without a lot of perspiration.[1]

Are you ready to sweat?

Getting your heart rate up is a great way to get sweating.

TARGET HEART RATES

A quick calculation to find your maximum target heart rate is to calculate 220 beats per minute (bpm) minus your age i.e. 220 – 49 years = 171 bpm.

During moderate intensity activities, your target heart rate is between 50-70% of the maximum heart rate, and vigorous activity is between 70-85% of the maximum heart rate. The below figures are averages; use them as a general guide.

AGE	beats per minute (bpm)	
	TARGET HEART RATE ZONE 50–85%	**AVERAGE MAXIMUM HEART RATE 100%**
20 years	100–170 bpm	200 bpm
30 years	95–162 bpm	190 bpm

35 years	93–157 bpm	185 bpm
40 years	90–153 bpm	180 bpm
45 years	88–149 bpm	175 bpm
50 years	85–145 bpm	170 bpm
55 years	83–140 bpm	165 bpm
60 years	80–136 bpm	160 bpm
65 years	78–132 bpm	155 bpm
70 years	75–128 bpm	150 bpm

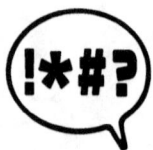

SWEAR

I'm convinced that swearing during exercise improves performance and helps you deal with the f#&king pain. Dr Richard Stephen at Keele University, UK, tested the effects of swearing on anaerobic power.

The researchers organised two experiments where 29 participants firstly underwent a test of anaerobic power on an exercise bike for a short, intense period of time without swearing, and then repeated this activity while being allowed to swear. Another test saw 52 participants complete an isometric handgrip test again with no swearing and then with swearing. In both cases, participants produced more power and strength if they swore![2]

It's about channelling that energy into something positive. Swearing is a great strategy if used in the right way. Be careful though, nobody likes a potty mouth!

SMILE

When we smile, we trick the brain that we're happy, triggering the release of the hormone cortisol as well as endorphins such as dopamine and serotonin that instantly lift your mood. When it comes to loading the squat rack, I smile and soldier on. It has worked for me so far as I'm squatting more than I ever have before.

In fact smiling isn't just for the weight workouts, research from the *Psychology of Sports and Exercise*, shows that smiling makes running easier and helps reduce muscle tension and distracts runners from uncomfortable body sensations.[3]

Using this 3 point system of **Sweat** — **Swear** — **Smile** will propel you to greater heights and I dare you to give it a go! I have created a quick reference guide that you can refer back to, to remind yourself of my personal philosophy. Feel free to add to it as you please and as you progress. For your quick reference guide, email me at info@leanmuscle.com with the subject line 'reference guide'.

SWEAT SWEAR SMILE

	PSYCHOLOGICALLY	PHYSICALLY	EMOTIONALLY
SWEAT	• Allows us to see the work is paying off making us feel good.	• Clears your body of heavy metals and chemicals. • Bacteria cleansing. • Boosts immunity. • Cools body down and regulates your body temperature. • Fights disease when feeling unwell.	• Gives us a sense of accomplishment. • Improves mood and sleep.

SWEAR	• Swearing enables us to go that bit extra.	• Activates the amygdala resulting in more power. • Elevates endorphins and serotonin levels. • Increases circulation. • Lowers pain levels.	• Overall sense of happiness and release, calmness and wellbeing.
SMILE	• Feel good factor. • Puts you in the moment and you connect with yourself. • Induces creativity (i.e. problem solving).	• Relaxes body and can lower heart rate and blood pressure. • Endorphins act as a natural pain reliever. • Boosts serotonin levels.	• Uplifts mood. • Boosts confidence and you smile more.

WHY I HAVE STOOD THE TEST OF TIME
AND LOVED BEING A PERSONAL TRAINER SINCE THE EARLY '80s

I have been so fortunate to find my purpose in life and wake every morning with a huge smile on my face knowing I am living my dream, that I found my true calling, even though it took time, mistakes and persistence.

Who knew that when I began training people in my 20s I would eventually make a living out of it? Back then it was never considered as a full-time career. I believe having a personal trainer is an essential service and everyone should find a personal trainer who is right for them, helping them stay on track with their health and fitness goals.

When I first commenced in the industry, only the wealthy and famous could afford to use personal trainers. Nowadays it is accessible to anyone and everyone who is serious about fitness or needing some help to make lifestyle changes.

I find great satisfaction in witnessing the change in someone's body, mood and life when they train with me. I love how it's more than just training — my clients confide in me, share their fears, cry with me, and I see how resilient they are (and they eventually see it in themselves).

I encourage and see them push beyond their limits to greater heights. And with that, the client feels they can achieve anything they set their mind to — it's empowering and inspiring to see. That connection is the difference.

A personal trainer should embody resilience, and they must be able to walk the talk. To this day I still push myself hard, training to achieve personal best results and I still love competing well into my 50s. I am at the forefront of my game and this gives me credibility and time-proven tools to work and share with my clients.

I've seen my fair share of trainers that don't gel with clients — their focus is either distracted, or on the 'mechanics' of training. When you are your authentic self and encourage your clients to laugh, share a joke or talk about the day, this is what makes the experience a great one; this is what clients remember — your encouragement and connection.

When clients decide to work with a personal trainer it often surprises me how little research they undertake. Quite often the fitness industry has been a one-size-fits-all approach, however for a small boutique gym like ours, the trend is returning to tailored training at a local gym or studio.

I believe the saying — you pay for what you get — holds true, especially in the personal training industry. When I see new clients I expect them to have done their research on the studio trainers, and have chosen to work with a trainer that specialises in the area they're aiming for. Having trainers niched in a specialty, enables the trainer to work to their strengths and not to be everything to everyone, and then the client gets the targeted results they're looking for.

Seeing a client's confidence grow as their body changes and the pride they feel when they reach their goals is the most rewarding moment for me. Sometimes it is hard to believe that they were once the shy, insecure, quiet, out of shape or depressed/unhappy person that first made contact with me to transform their body, mind and entire being a few months before. It takes courage for someone to admit they need help and it's something I never take for granted.

A STRONG BODY SAVED MY LIFE...
IT COULD SAVE YOURS ONE DAY TOO

It was February 2020 and I had just finished a gruelling arm session at the gym and then jumped on my electric pushbike for my 30-minute ride home. I rode everywhere, I loved the feeling and clarity a bike ride induced, especially during peak hour traffic where there was the feeling of being streets ahead in life.

But this day was different. I was travelling around 30km per hour (which feels faster on a bike than the safe confines of a car) and the next thing I knew, I was laying on the ground across the tram tracks in the middle of the road. They say your life flashes before your eyes in moments of trauma — I'll agree it happened to me.

I was in shock and immobile as bystanders gathered around. They stopped traffic to handle the situation until the emergency services arrived. They tried to gently explain what had happened and reassure me of where I was and that I had no broken limbs or deep wounds. My first instinct was to make sure my expensive electric bike was okay — Danni had just bought this for me for my 54th birthday.

I felt badly bruised and was holding my ribs with snot dribbling down my chest but I was alive.

The lady that had 'car-doored' me called an ambulance; wanting to make sure I had no internal injuries. Apart from being in shock, I was stable. By the time the ambulance arrived my family were on the scene.

Having never needed an ambulance before in my life, I was reluctant at first but eventually persuaded to take a trip to the hospital, and then given painkillers. On the ride to the hospital the ambulance officer asked for my particulars, including my age. He had a look of shock on his face when I told him my age as he had thought I was in my mid 30s.

After a thorough check, the doctor advised I was fortunate to have no internal injuries. I believe my physique certainly softened the blow and that having muscle is not only functional but lifesaving! I had never really viewed my health this way.

The moral of this story is that weight training is not only about feeling great and looking fit; it's also about preventing yourself from serious injury. The body is a smart and incredible machine and we often take that for granted. I truly feel if it were not for my level of fitness, I could have been writing this chapter from a hospital bed or not at all! My muscle thickness gave me internal strength to withstand the impact of the collision, and my years of training had given me mental toughness to recover quickly from the accident too.

SWEAT SWEAR SMILE

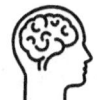

CHAPTER 2

MINDSET IS EVERYTHING

I have three pillars of philosophy behind a successful fitness journey: training, mindset and nutrition. Each part is as important as the other but I believe the most important place to begin is with mindset. They say winning isn't everything but I say wanting to *is*.

Your attitude going into any challenge often determines your outcome, but have you ever wondered where your attitude comes from? Growing up with a twin equally as competitive as I played a big part in creating my never-give-up attitude.

Tony and I were always competing against each other, pushing ourselves and doing whatever it took to win. Sometimes we won; sometimes we lost. I recall one tough game of footy when we were young, Tony had been pretty confident he would take out Best On Ground, but that day I took the title. Tony elbowed me in the ribs all the way home in the back seat of Dad's Volkswagen. I took the pain and rubbed it in even more – this was our constant competitiveness and today, we laugh and joke about it.

Imagining that moment of winning was a huge force behind our persistence and determination to keep going even after getting beaten. Eventually this would pay off in our individual achievements, we just had to hang in there. Tony's tenacity was unbelievable, it's what enabled him to launch himself fearlessly into a pack of much larger footy players and he'd be the one to emerge from between them all with the ball in his hands.

Back then I didn't understand 'how' I reached my goal; I just kept envisioning the result I wanted in my mind. I constantly remind my clients (and myself) that visualisation is the way to plant ideas and goals into your subconscious mind and a healthy way to create your own, personal vision statement. It's a matter of simply closing your eyes, using your imagination, and mentally creating the pictures in your mind, like running a movie of your desired results on repeat. This will then become the reality in your subconscious and replaying it with emotion will help you to change old habits and increase performance.

This is not a new technique and has been around for centuries. There are so many ways to use visualisation. It has been used in the field of sports psychology and personal development to increase stamina, reach personal and professional goals, and exceed any limits the athlete may have had before.

'Goal Visualisation' is common with athletes across the globe and simply means that in their minds' eye they can already see themselves having achieved their goal, whether it be the desired body they are aiming for, or the ideal lifting weight or competing and winning in their chosen field.

From the words of a special teacher and friend who once told me,

> "Fred, the use of mental imagery is one of the strongest and most effective strategies for making something happen for you."
>
> — *Dr Wayne Dyer*

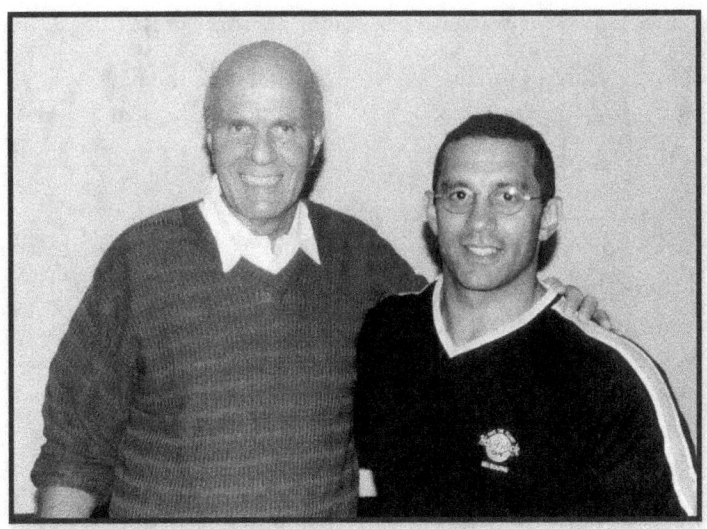

I have never forgotten that advice. My wish to meet Dr Wayne Dyer came true after reading many of his books (my favourite being *The Power of Intention*). I listened with great interest and intent when he presented a series of seminars in Sydney in 2001. Wayne's talks on stage about how your thoughts are your currency really ignited the possibility in me that I could create the life I imagined and not give in to the opinions of others. I could feel my worth, which focused my attention on my dreams in a positive way.

The best way I can think of honouring him is to live his teachings, to realise who we are deep inside and, "to see the light in others," as he often said. As well as urging everyone to help lift humanity to the frequency of joy, love, decency and kindness.

Thank you Dr Wayne Dyer, for touching my soul and the souls of many, for empowering us to live our best lives.

> *"Strength does not come from winning. Your struggles develop your strengths. When you go through hardships and decide not to surrender, that is strength."*
>
> *— Arnold Schwarzenegger*

Meeting Arnold Schwarzenegger taught me some great rules to live by:

1. Don't be afraid to fail
2. Break some rules
3. Trust yourself
4. Ignore the naysayers
5. Work like hell
6. Give back

His other advice was to figure out what makes you happy, no matter how crazy it sounds to other people.

It's time for you to do that now and analyse your own mindset.

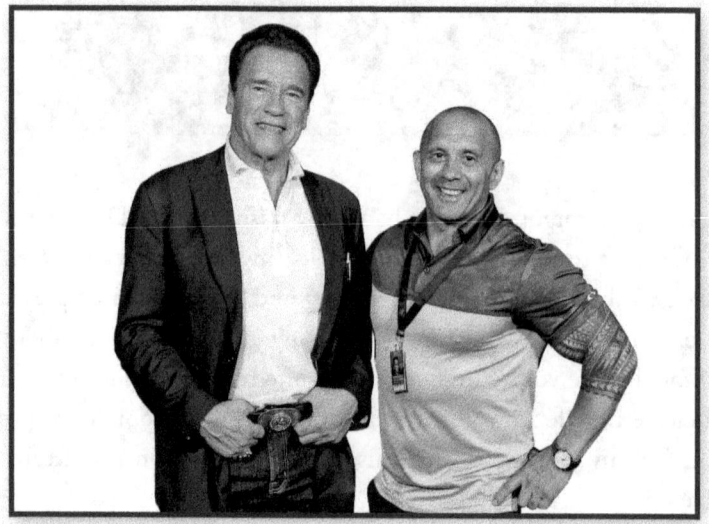

What is your current mindset towards your body, health and fitness? How do you feel about your ability to achieve your goals in this moment? Optimistic or overwhelmed?

....

....

....

....

....

Now describe your future vision for yourself, how you want to be, feel or look. Let yourself imagine the feeling of reaching that goal.

Look for words from someone who inspires you, to go the extra distance to achieve your goal, to be the best you can be. Think of those words as you train, they can have a huge affect on your mindset and motivation.

WILLPOWER – A USELESS WORD

As a personal trainer, the number one reason why people contact me is because they can't achieve their fitness goals alone, they come to me for guidance and support, which is a courageous first step. I have seen so many people 'try' to lose weight purely on willpower. They think it's all about how much weight they can lose and how quickly.

They're usually hooked on some promise of a magic pill or a late night infomercial selling a product that manipulates them with unrealistic images about getting your body back. Even if they manage to lose some weight, they will typically gain it all back, often more than before. I tell them using willpower is as bad as doing nothing. Let me explain.

The first problem here is that willpower is only a conscious undertaking; it is superficial and easily loses any ground it might make. Your minute-to-minute and day-to-day choices are usually guided by your *sub*conscious mind, not the conscious mind, so you will always default back to your subconscious motivations.

If I have lost you here stay with me. The subconscious mind functions below the surface of our awareness and activates whenever a sequence of thoughts, words or events take place. The subconscious mind controls our beliefs, behaviours, habits and even the words we say. It also contains the foundation of how these thoughts and actions started, possibly back when we were children. It operates on really old programming and can undermine all our efforts.

If we do not try to unravel the reasons why we sabotage ourselves, we continue this pattern of not fulfilling the promises we make to ourselves, we give up early and we end up doing what we swore to ourselves we wouldn't do. This could be choosing to have ice-cream instead of doing those sit-ups we had planned. Sound familiar? Our subconscious minds want to satisfy our immediate desire which sabotages our long-term desire. Imagine the power if you change your thoughts, you can change your life!

There is a bigger reason why willpower is useless – our subconscious motivations are more powerful than our consciousness; they learn, hold and efficiently recall frequently used behaviour patterns. So our healthy, conscious desires are not only outnumbered, they're outmanoeuvred. Willpower is useless as a weight loss tool, because it puts you at war with yourself and unfortunately, it's a war you can't win as long as your self-sabotaging motivations remain unchanged.

Awareness of these motivations is the first step to changing them. I'll start easy on you ☺, be honest with your answers without criticising yourself. It is brave to acknowledge your very human imperfections and even braver to try to better yourself. Now is the time to face unhelpful thoughts and habits and move forward.

Can you identity any self-sabotaging behaviours? Procrastinating? Stress-eating? Constant excuses?

Can you identify any thoughts that are holding you back from real change? Old thoughts that feel like the 'truth' but in fact are simply beliefs from a deep part of your programming?

....

....

....

....

....

....

....

....

I know I am making some pretty strong assertions here about just how 'programmed' we really are without knowing it. However, think how our subconscious mind continuously operates our physical bodies such as our heartbeat, breathing and circulation, and it does all of this without any conscious thought from us, it's simply part of our survival biology.

Likewise our subconscious mind controls our verbal and physical actions and reactions based on our past experiences that tell us, 'This is how we survived last time.' But today is about thriving, not just surviving! The subconscious mind likes doing familiar things so breaking those cycles is often challenging, but so life changing.

Do you wish to spend your days at the mercy of your subconscious that mechanically reacts to the external forces happening *to* you? Going along with this programming and the old familiar places it takes you? It will feel same old same old as long as you let it. Often we become part of the ebb and flow of other people's decisions in our lives too, and we are left trying to justify how we came to reach a destination that was not our own.

Have you ever looked back and wondered how on earth you became so involved in something that you didn't really feel strongly about? Chances are you were flowing along in someone else's current.

Jim Rohn, respected American entrepreneur summed up this passive life strategy perfectly when he said: *"If you don't design your own life plan, chances are you'll fall into someone else's plan. And guess what they have planned for you? Not much."*

Are you ready to live a life that is healthier, happier and works for you? So stop being the victim of what life throws at you, acknowledge what's happening, question it to gain a greater awareness of your options, then consciously *choose* a path that will create and generate a greater life according to your own priorities and goals.

Let's use the concept of programming to your advantage. You can change your thoughts and change your life by looking closely at each self-sabotaging behaviour you identified in the previous exercise by asking yourself:

When this self-sabotaging behaviour occurs, what is it you feel or sense? Do you recognise it as unhelpful behaviour yet do it anyway?

....

....

....

....

....

....

....

....

....

What do you say to yourself the moment you feel it, in that split second of awareness before your consciousness filters it?

....

....

....

....

....

....

What can you do differently next time you notice yourself going down the same limited path? How can you jump tracks and create a new positive, conscious thought and action plan?

....

....

....

....

....

....

Going through this exercise helps you leave the old programming and jump to your new improved program. You may not get it right on the first attempt, or even the second. With anything, you will succeed with practice, patience and persistence. These are known as the three P's of success. Remember each step builds on the last and you'll reach the big goal you're asking for sooner than you think.

I know that you *can* do it, but *will* you do it?

Do not let anyone stop you or tell you that you're not enough. You are absolutely good enough and if you need a hand I'm here to help you achieve that goal. It's my purpose.

A big challenge we face in Australia is that of the 'tall poppy' syndrome. If you're unfamiliar with the term, it refers to knocking down someone who has risen above others in their field to achieve success. It stems back to the Aussie idea of everyone being given a 'fair go' but nowadays many people see other's success as a threat or a reminder that they are not achieving their own success.

If my brother had listened to the critics who claimed he couldn't succeed as an AFL player because of his short stature, it's fair to say he probably wouldn't have succeeded to the extent he did. He succeeded because he didn't listen to anyone except his own voice, his own vision. On the field, Tony was even known to intimidate much taller players; it's all in your mindset. Stay true to your dream and let everything else fall away.

There may be people around you who try to bring you down — to make themselves feel better — those 'so-called' friends will continue to try to put you back into your rabbit hole and want you to conform back to who you used to be, the person *they* are used to. My advice is to just let them be, let them go and get back to making changes and focusing on your goals.

These people may slip away or become not-so-close friends, but that's okay because this makes room for those who have your back. You can do it and you can begin right now — nothing is stopping you!

Even if you run into problems along the way, know that you can get past them, with effort and with help, you're helping yourself already by reading this book. No matter how big or small your goal is, you can do it. It just requires determination, effort, as well as a strong commitment and persistence. I encourage you to take your success to the next level by working with a personal trainer who will not only keep you accountable but also be an all-round positive influence helping you achieve your goals.

The physical shape and fitness that I work to maintain and enjoy today are living proof that the right attitude can manifest any dream.

CONQUERING FEAR

Rather than something real, I like to think of this feeling as False Evidence Appearing Real (FEAR). Often it is uncertainty or fear of the unknown that is the real issue. Fear of something you've never tried before. It holds so many people back from starting their fitness journey or taking it to the next level. They ask themselves, "Can I really do it?" or "What if I fail?"

These are natural questions but fear is not there to stop you; it's there to help you assess the risk and prepare yourself.

Remember you can't fail; it just means the journey isn't over yet.

Fear can be a really positive tool to use. Did you know fear and excitement feel exactly the same in your body? I invite you next time you feel fearful to ask yourself, "Is this actual fear or excitement?" If it's excitement, you've got an extra kick to push past your limitations.

I also learned long ago the only way to get beyond your fear is to power right through it. If you practise performing the thing you fear, then the fear loses its control over you. *Do it to lose it.* Let's say that again…***Do it to lose it!***

Have you ever seen the comedian Bob Newhart's skit on counselling fear? In a nutshell he frankly tells his clients they must, "Stop it!" None of their excuses matter, he just insists they can stop it if they concentrate. His advice gets the job done and saves time and worry. It reminds us how simple it is to change something when we respond consciously.

There are some fears that are justifiable in the beginning, like going into your very first bodybuilding competition (which was really excitement anyway) but other fears are only roadblocks put there by yourself and your old programming. Regardless of how valid you think the fear is, there is never a good reason for it to control you or your situation. Over the years when competing, I learned to become fearless, embracing it and stepping onto the stage. My nickname became Fearless Freddie.

In saying this, it is important to always look ahead before moving forward. You want to assess the risks, do you have support or are you prepared to go it alone? Then armed with knowledge and preparation, tread carefully as you move forward. Confidence, ability, strength and success are not built by seeking refuge in what is comfortable and familiar, they are built by venturing into unknown territory, prepared for the challenges and determined to do whatever is necessary. This is about finding the courage and self-motivation in us all.

Let the fear sharpen your awareness, and then let it inspire you to act. Fear shows how important your goal really is to you. On the other side of fear is the achievement you seek.

HONOURING THE JOURNEY
KNOWING YOUR 'WHAT-WHY-HOW'

It may sound like a cliché, but understanding and respecting your vision holds true especially when undergoing a fitness campaign. Building a body that can move you from maintenance to progress each day is my mantra; progress literally comes down to 'one rep' at a time. Remember a strong body gives you every chance for good health as you age, which is an amazing incentive.

For someone like me in his 50s, getting into tiptop shape and staying in shape is a lot like a build project. First, there must be a clear vision in mind ('what') and you must know and understand your motivation for the vision ('why') then the vision goes onto paper as a blueprint ('how') and finally comes the execution of all these elements of your 'what-why-how'. If you don't have these three things, chances are your goal will just be a dream stuck on repeat and failing you each time.

Let's break down the 'what-why-how' of your journey further. The 'what' of your goal is a straightforward statement. It's a clear description of your dream, what is the finish line of your goal? For example one of my past dreams was winning the bodybuilding title of Mr Australasia.

The 'why' is all about your motivation behind your dream, why you are doing it. If this answer isn't clear or you're not 100% honest with yourself, you will remain on the merry-go-round of weight loss.

For example, it was a boyhood dream of mine to win a major title, to reach the height of achievement in the industry I loved. But I was also driven to achieve this because I knew getting to number 1 accorded credibility and authority in the industry through becoming the best bodybuilder I could be; it's a competitive industry where 2nd place isn't so often remembered. This achievement would help give standing, integrity and longevity in the industry I loved.

The 'how' is all about the practicalities of achieving your goal and what resources you will tap into.

- Will you engage the services of a personal trainer?
- Will you get the support of your loved-ones helping to keep you accountable?
- How often are you going to train?
- What diet changes are you willing to make? How will you prepare your meals? If you don't plan ahead, complacency, tiredness and impatience could see you reach for easy, unsuitable choices.
- How will you get your mind in order to really catapult your success? Tackling that unconscious mind is often a big part of your 'how'.

Before I began preparing for my title competition and also for my own 12-Week Challenges in the past, I have engaged in a Personal Trainer for myself. We would sit down and clearly map out a plan of attack and I would then be accountable to him each week for the training I undertook.

I admit I have had another amazing resource in my life to add to my 'how': Danni. Having the support of a close family member can be a real game-changer. They can become your biggest supporter, provide unbiased feedback and stop you from opening the fridge every five minutes!

Many times I have opened a discussion with Danni about my latest goal and she has offered her support in wonderful ways. She distracts me from looking for food unnecessarily, reminds me to go to bed early, calls me out on my bad habits, prepares my clothes for my workouts and often prepares the right meals for my training (believe me, I know how lucky I am!).

She makes sure I do my low impact cardio like going for a walk and in return I give her foot massages (play it smart and the results can be a win/win situation ☺). It's a stark fact that training can be tough and your moods occasionally get affected, but it's really important to be kind to yourself and those around you.

So once you know your 'what', think long and hard to work out the important 'why' and 'how' parts to your goal, have a clear process and the journey will honour you back tenfold. It might take time; your dream developing slowly until you can't take one more day of the old you and your determination will win out!

NOTHING HAPPENS STRAIGHT AWAY

The truth is it can take a few weeks to lay the foundation of your new routine and habits, and it's hard to accept that even more hard work and soul searching awaits you. You see, each moment of the day is part of the journey even if it doesn't seem like much is happening.

Sometimes you feel you are going backwards instead of forwards, that particular week is a struggle because you are not seeing what you want straight away, it feels harder and more difficult than you imagined it to be; this is when you — *keep going!*

The mirror may be showing you a reflection of what you saw yesterday, and that's okay, but *know* that one day it will all come together, then BANG! Suddenly, you begin to see the small improvements around your body and evidence of your hard work and persistence is starting to show itself.

Stay the course and one day soon, you'll see pieces of that blueprint you wrote down at the start manifest right before your eyes, staring back at you in the mirror. It is a moment people remember for a long time, the beginning of real change.

My realisation of that exact process occurred when I was aiming to achieve the body of a Mr Australia amateur bodybuilder. It didn't happen overnight, it took time, patience and a lot of trial and error (on my part) to get it right. Oftentimes it felt like nothing was happening until one day, it just did, and on that day I was so grateful I didn't give up, instead nurturing my goal and persisting with the training, remaining focused and repeatedly visualising.

I know after being in the game for four decades that growth and development of any kind always requires a gestation period, a bit like the anticipation of a baby's arrival. An expectant mother would not hurry the process because she knows every minute of the pregnancy the baby is developing essential bones and cells for its growth in preparation to function in the world on its own. Look at your body in this way too. If you ever get frustrated with the rate of progress with your fitness (and most people do), just remember that success is *always* guaranteed to those who are persistent.

I can become impatient for results at times too so once a week, I check in with my own personal trainer who continues to remind me that, "It just takes time Fred."

I like to think that you can become like Michelangelo and be the architect and builder of your own dream body. Trust me when I tell you that you will build the body you want and eventually, if you are patient enough and refuse to quit, you will be able to tell others the secret of how you did it too. Set your goals high, create that blueprint and keep going.

> *"The greatest danger for most of us lies in not setting our aim too high and falling short; but in setting our aim too low, and achieving our mark."*
>
> *— Michelangelo*

I understand you may feel some goals are unrealistic, but the way I see it, the goals themselves are not unrealistic; it is the deadline that makes them so. Anything is possible if you give it enough time.

Keep laying those 'reps' every day, one at a time, and sure enough you will build yourself your own dream body.

THE RIGHT SPACE TO FOCUS

Your training time will become a mental workout, focusing your breathing and energy in each moment, in deep concentration or the zone state. You can think of your gym (even if it's in your garage at home) as though it is a sacred space, a dedicated space to concentrate on your goal, letting everything else in your life fade away.

Don't cut corners here thinking a 3m x 3m space in the living room will cut it. Casually wandering over to a small corner of your room to try and work out just won't hone your concentration to connect with your muscles and get you in the right state of mind to push yourself. You need to honour your workout space and invest in it wisely.

One thing I know holds true (a lesson from my twin), is that wherever you find that sacred place, approach it with 'white line fever'. This means as soon as you cross the entry point to that space, you're no longer distracted by the outside world. This is all about giving it your all. Even when I train on my own or with a trainer, I often go to another gym because I know my studio can be a distraction. I make a point to go to a different environment so I can focus.

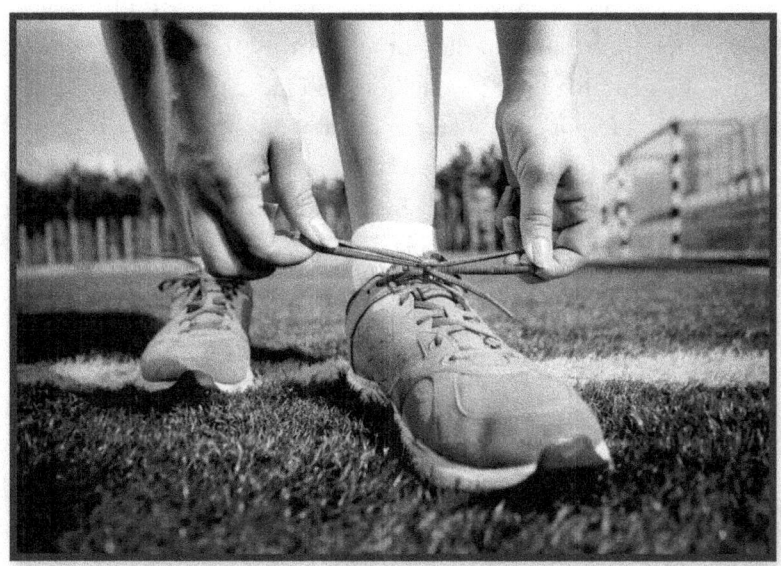

You need a space dedicated to training, where you can focus, push yourself, hone your abilities, reflect on your workout to improve upon, and progress towards your goal. Bottom line is, I've always loved the mental zone of physical training whatever the environment, and I have chosen to make it a habit and an important part of my everyday life!

I love how the benefits of training overflow into other areas. I have found learning new skills and techniques, focusing on each phase of movement and following through, supporting this foundation with nutrition and regular practising of all of the above, has not only helped me to lift weights but improved every facet of my life in the form of better self-control, discipline and work ethic.

Exercise has been shown time and time again to increase your overall health. Not only can exercise be fun and social, regular exercise helps combat health conditions and diseases, controls weight, improves bone strength, improves mood, boosts energy and promotes better sleep. All this gives you the best preparation for a long, healthy life.

Lift, learn, connect as best you can and then repeat the process again and again. Be sure to go at your own pace, take things slow, but more importantly continue to push yourself to be a better athlete than you were the day before, then the month and year before that. Often when I witness people embarking on their fitness journey they let their stories get in their way, doubting their own abilities and judgement, such as "I'm not a runner," or, "I'm not coordinated enough."

I can help you push past those fake stories and find ways that you can do it to suit your level. It's a limitation you've created to keep you where you are; safe and comfortable. But you can still feel secure as you s-t-r-e-t-c-h and grow if you have the right preparation and guidance to realise your vision.

For example, one of my clients, Rebecca told me vehemently, "I'm not a runner, I will never be a runner." I challenged her on that fake story running through her brain because the truth is she had never tried.

I asked her if she could run for 30 seconds, she said she could. She started off running in 30-second intervals and walked for 10-minutes in between, for a total of 45 minutes. Over time we slowly increased that original 30-seconds to 1 minute, and then 2 minutes, then 5 minutes and so on. Before too long Rebecca was running 8–10kms and within the year she decided to train for a half-marathon. Not bad for someone who was convinced they weren't a runner and *never* could be.

It's important to challenge your fake stories and not just automatically believe something because it may have been true in your childhood. By challenging our beliefs and fake stories, we make room for new stories and experiences to appear.

CRUSHING YOUR LIMITATIONS

We've spoken about tall poppy syndrome, but what about the inner monologue of critique that goes on in our head every day? Sometimes it's subtle and fleeting, but nonetheless it's there. It's time to kick that 'itty-bitty-shitty' committee to the curb! Talking to yourself when training either drives you to achieve more or stops you in your tracks. To stop the vicious cycle, let's rephrase the way we talk. Aside from using the positive language and self-talk that you know about, I'm going to challenge and shift your mindset.

When you ask yourself a question with an answer already in mind, your answer only recalls what you know and you're likely to be hoping the answer will validate your current position. If you rephrase your question, you gain a different awareness to other possibilities (i.e. how to raise the bar) and leads to asking yourself other questions that cut through to the hard-hitting honest answers.

I encourage you to ask open-ended questions *without* an answer at the ready. Instead of starting a question passively with the words how or why, rephrase it to something like this, "What would it take to …?" This makes you workshop outside the box to get a *different* answer.

So if you ask yourself, "What would it take to create extra time in my day to train?" You have to give yourself a tough, solid answer such as, "I will have to wake up an hour earlier to train before work," or "I will have to start work earlier so I can leave work earlier to train." This is the reality of your dream starting to take shape. You won't change if nothing changes in your life.

Be proactive and specific in your questions, "What would it take to do one more rep? What would it take to beat my personal best?" This unconsciously issues a challenge to yourself that fires your body up to achieve one more!

> *"If you really want to do something, you'll find a way. If you don't, you'll find an excuse."*
>
> — *Jim Rohn*

EMPOWERED TO SAY NO

If you really want to achieve your goal, then changes need to be made to create time each day and to create space in your mind to achieve your goal.

Saying no is empowering. It helps you stay true to your priorities. You can focus on you for a change and ultimately you feel better. It can also lead to opportunities to say yes with a clear head; saying no can create space where there wasn't any before.

Remember it's okay to say no if something doesn't work for you, an invitation or agreeing to favours too often that eat into your training time. It's okay to say no to that extra helping or piece of cake. And it's okay to say no without giving a reason – we often feel obliged to explain our answer if it's no.

THE POWER OF SILENCE

There is another tool in my toolkit that has been an integral part of my learning and success over the years. It might surprise you but the simple act of sitting in silence can really focus your day and increase your output.

I have always practised meditation even before I knew what the benefits were. Perhaps it was an extension of my Catholic upbringing but each morning I would close my eyes and let the universe tell me which way to go, where I should be. It helped to quieten the inner noise of my mind that kept wrestling with my young ego in every situation.

It helped to carry me more calmly through the day.

Meditation brings your brainwave patterns into an alpha state, which promotes healing. Afterwards the mind is instantly refreshed. Meditation can help in clearing away any build-up of stress, clears away those thoughts stuck on repeat and it helps in eliminating negative self talk.

From my studies into anatomy and physiology, this led me into the study of the mind and I came across the teachings of Deepak Chopra and Eckhart Tolle, their philosophies really connected with my thought process. You can't expect different results thinking with the same mind that created the old results.

Sitting in stillness allows you to reflect on your thoughts with more simplicity and clarity; it connects you with something deeper and solidifies your decisions and goals. The universe is there for us in its infinite wisdom and connecting with it is an important part of my day. Getting up twenty minutes earlier in the morning and just being in silence gives me a sense of power each day. It's a gift that keeps on giving. Best of all you don't have to be a guru to do it; it requires very little practice and is a powerful approach to life and seeing your dreams to fruition.

Some of the benefits to meditating every day include:
- Gaining a new perspective on stressful situations
- Building skills to manage stress
- Increasing self-awareness
- Better focus on the present
- Reducing negative emotions
- Improving sleep
- Increasing air flow to the body
- Improving blood flow
- And so many other physical benefits as well

Most of the people I meet on their quest to fitness come with some sort of physical pain and discomfort yet they do not realise some of it is due to the inner dialogue happening in their minds. I like to remind my clients it is important they work from the inside out which will help them understand their situation a whole lot clearer.

Everyone has a story they tell themselves that either stops them from getting what they want or propels them to move towards it.

I like to get you thinking by asking, **"What does your story do for you?"**

It is difficult to change your story but meditation can help restructure your sense of purpose and commitment to be the best you can be starting from the inside.

We all have greatness within us but first we have to find and commit to our own set of 'non-negotiables' (our 'why') and as our desire grows so does our refusal for compromise – we'll do whatever it takes to have or be whatever we desire. Through meditating daily, I reconnect with my goal.

Check out my Introduction to Meditation audio at leanmuscle.com.

When you join the 12-Week Challenge you'll receive a 30-minute meditation audio to listen to daily.

A REAL GAME PLAN

So do you have a real game plan?

The purpose of this book is to help build your foundation to go after and achieve the goal you set. Whether it's better health, better fitness, a toned body, lean muscle, lifting weights or losing weight, you need a game plan. It's one thing to think it or say it out loud, but without a written game plan, how will you achieve it? Life is short and regret is a bitch so stop waiting!

Let's get down and dirty and get that game plan on the page.

What is it you desire to achieve? Be specific.

....
....
....
....
....
....
....

Why do you want to achieve this goal? Why does it light you up?

....
....
....
....
....
....
....

Where are you now? List what's holding you back, the limitations of your inner dialogue.

When you achieve your goal, what does that look and feel like to you in six months' time? Is it more energy to play with the kids in the backyard or aiming to lift a certain weight?

How will you achieve your goal? What resources will you need? Make sure you block out time daily for the next 12 weeks.

....
....
....
....
....
....
....
....

What do you need to change? Nutrition, mindset, sleep?

....
....
....
....
....
....
....

When would you like to achieve this by?

Who will be your support crew?

What action can you take to motivate yourself when you don't feel like training or find yourself steering off track?

....
....
....
....
....
....
....
....

What mini goals can you aim for to demonstrate you're moving closer to your goal? Remember you're playing the long game – lasting changes take time.

....
....
....
....
....
....
....
....

What can you say no to, to help you reach your goal?

....
....
....
....
....
....

Once you reach your goal, what's next? When you get better, the game gets bigger.

....
....
....
....
....
....
....
....

Make sure you finish this crucial step before turning the page. You might have to sacrifice things you've been used to doing for a long time. Believe me, it's necessary and may keep happening as your goal draws closer. I encourage you to update your answers as you move through the book.

We can all dream bigger and create more impact than we ever thought possible. Part of my life's mission has been to inspire and ignite people into the greatness within them and create a meaningful life every day. It gets me up early in the morning and lights a fire under my step each and every day.

DISCIPLINE

A game plan is one thing but having the discipline to execute it to the letter is another. As an amateur bodybuilder that has successfully competed in my 20s, 30s, 40s and 50s, I have found discipline to be the most powerful, most important tool to master. For me, discipline is nothing more than controlling my own behaviour. This could include getting up early to train or preparing my meals in advance. Each moment of the day you're making decisions that contribute to your discipline. As you progress, your sense of discipline will start to overtake those sabotaging behaviours.

When it comes to transforming your body, I encourage you to be curious, ask questions, test and measure, and remember success leaves clues for you to follow. Hint: they usually refer back to tweaking your nutrition, mindset and training. I have always looked at successful people whose behaviour inspires me, and used their success as a model to learn from.

Just like those bodybuilders in the magazines I devoured all those years ago, I would study their model and strategies endlessly, breaking them down into small steps and then I'd rebuild them in a way that suited my body and my circumstances and resources at the time.

Without discipline I would never have achieved everything I have. For example one of my 'non-negotiables' was never to consume alcohol. I had never grown a taste for it plus my time as a bouncer when I was 20, taught me firsthand the poison it can be to people, I saw no goals were reached using alcohol.

It has been my relationships along the way, my memories, my fitness and the trophies in my cabinet that have become my reminders that discipline is always worth it. Remember, the real work of success takes place behind the scenes.

FOUR DECADES AND COUNTING

Learning discipline takes time I know. When I was young I had all the enthusiasm you could ask for. Although it was often misdirected it was never a wasted effort, it was a lesson. This is how I learnt the advantage of testing and measuring each method or technique. When something didn't work for me, I acknowledged, readjusted and tried again. I still apply this philosophy today.

I first entered competition bodybuilding in my early 20s to measure my potential as a weight trainer and to boost my confidence. I soon learnt the benefits of posing for muscle awareness and definition; improving my mind to muscle connection was a way to take my training to the next level and posing certainly helped my confidence.

I achieved many memorable highlights and wins in my career thanks to the value of learning consistency and patience in my three pillars of training, nutrition and mindset. From modest beginnings, the following images show the gradual and consistent results I have achieved over my four decades (and counting) in the world of fitness.

AS A TEEN

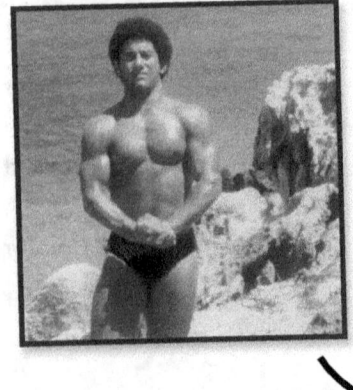

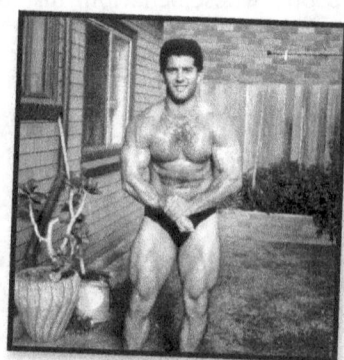

IN MY 20s

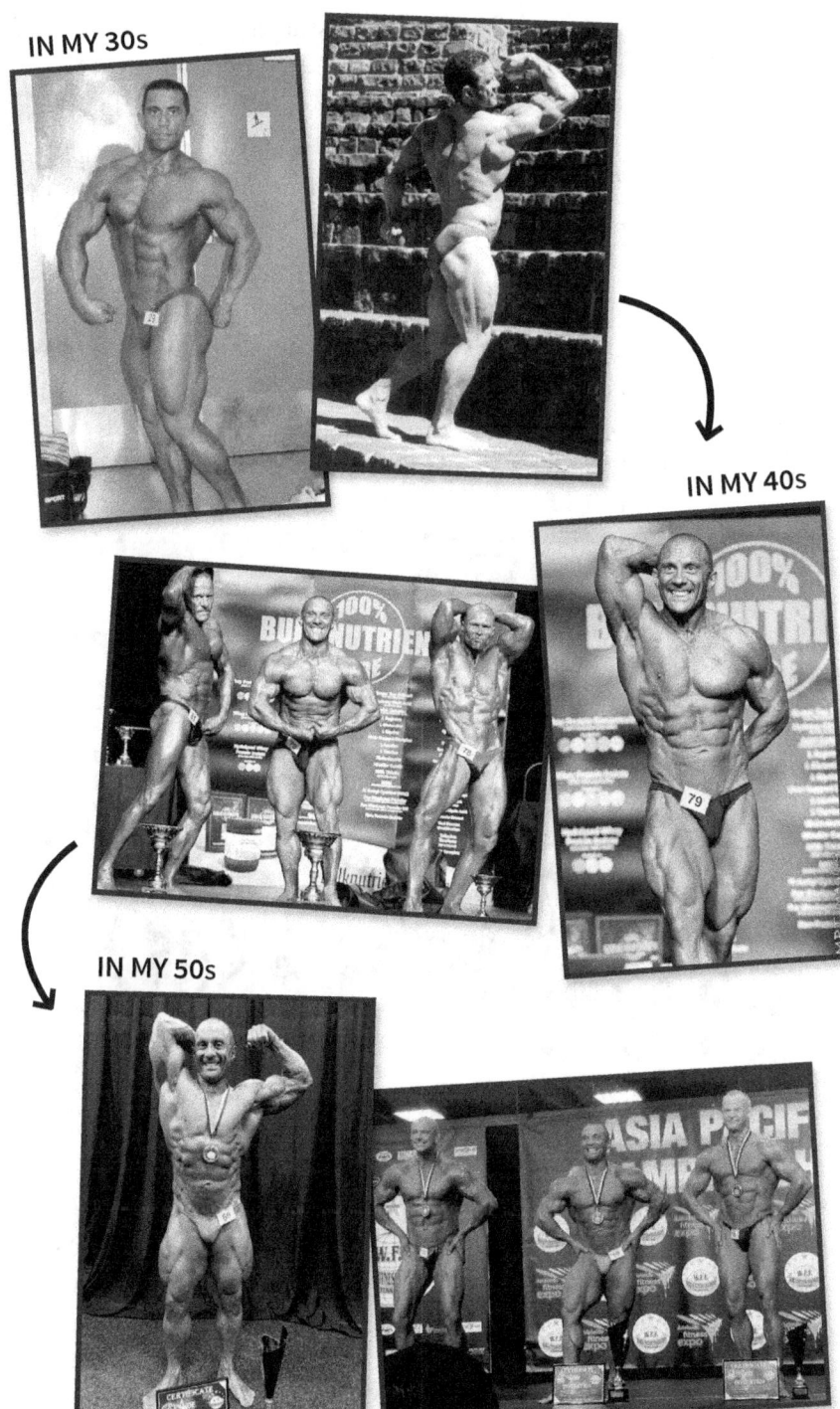

Fitness is an ongoing commitment that is never retired from. I need to be reminded of this occasionally and following my last win in 2016, I let my fitness slip somewhat, not deliberately, but I had let life get in the way – always 'busy'. I was running two studios at the time, eating quickly between clients, not paying attention to the fuel I was feeding my body, and I became complacent. I realised I had stopped walking my talk and decided enough was enough!

So at age 53 I underwent my own transformation. I took action and engaged a trainer, weighing in each week, sending in photos (yes I was accountable to my coach), paying attention to what I ate, shifting my mindset and sharing my vision. The work and persistence paid off, my health and energy levels were recharged and I felt new again.

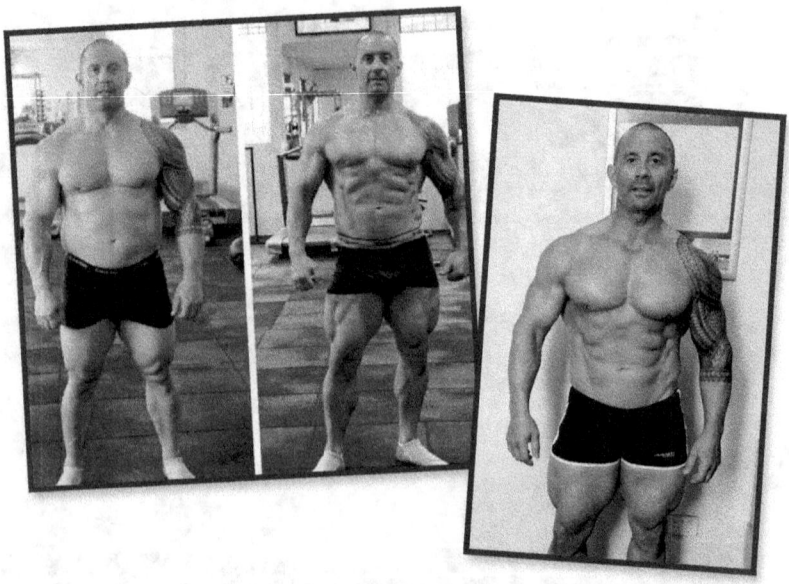

Besides the obvious physical improvement, putting myself in the clients' shoes was such a great lesson to remind me of the importance of my three pillars of training, mindset and nutrition. Now every year I personally complete a 12-Week Challenge, and I am working toward competing in my 60s. Training every day as though you have a competition coming up can really keep you on track.

NO MORE EXCUSES

Once you are clear on your what-why-how and have your game plan mapped out, you can move your training from maintenance (stagnant) to progression and tap into your goals daily or whenever you find yourself not putting the effort in.

Many people will look to personal trainers for answers when the real answers are already within them. All you need to do is ask questions, be honest with yourself about how much you are willing to put in and change. Your personal trainer is your guide to assist you, keep you on track and facilitate your progression. They can't give you all the answers and do the work for you. They'll give you plenty of options and structure to your game plan.

I have found structure is important to maintaining training motivation and that doing the hard stuff first sets you up nicely for the day. I like to train first thing in the morning as it elevates your energy for whatever your day holds. Establishing a routine and having excellent time and money management is also critical to remaining focused on the end result.

In order to amplify your goals, you must first address time, money and attitude. Personal training is a way to keep you accountable for your health and keep you on track toward your goals. This industry holds a lot of flaky promises, so it's important that you look at fitness as a lifestyle.

When a client states they cannot afford my program I answer them with a simple question, "Compared to what?" Your greatest asset is *you*, so why wouldn't you invest in your health and fitness? Never let money be an obstacle to your health. This is something I work out with my clients at the beginning of their training program so that it does not become a problem half way through.

There are options to suit all budgets: face-to-face, group training or online training. I have found once you have skin in the game (paying upfront) you have made a tangible commitment and you will be more motivated to work harder to fulfil your goals of weight loss and strength.

ACCOUNTABILITY

Let's face it, getting in shape is a massive task! If you have made the decision to *really* change your life, it's now time to take responsibility and make that change happen with my 12-Week Challenge program. It will give you the support and knowledge to get started and maintain a healthy lifestyle, and by taking on new tools and a new mindset, you'll benefit from new awareness and insights into other aspects of your life.

I know from personal experience it can be fearful and challenging to start something you know will change your life, please know I'll be with you every step of the way to keep you on track and accountable. When you are held accountable, you are less likely to cheat yourself out of the right foods, skip a class or workout. You have invested in yourself and you want to make sure you gain a ten-fold return on your investment. However, this requires work.

Accountability to me is a two-way street. My accountability as the trainer is to provide support and solutions to anything that may come up, and equip you with the tools and education to confidently take control of your own fitness goals. Once we start seeing results, the rewards are incredible. You will feel stronger, more in control and see that change really is possible. New potential is unlocked and a new mindset is formed, it's a very exciting development in your life. It takes time, but it's worth it and we are both accountable for creating success in your life.

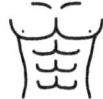

CHAPTER 3

BODY

BODY TYPES

Let's get down to details to understand the factors that can affect your results even before you begin. For any training and nutrition program, it's a good idea to know your somatotype – your natural shape and size.

There are three body types you are predisposed to fall under:
- Endomorph
- Mesomorph
- Ectomorph

Even within these categories, you can be a combination of two rather than a single type. Your genes, ethnicity, diet and exercise can influence your body type. Working with your body type (rather than against it) helps you create the healthiest, happiest and fittest you, naturally.

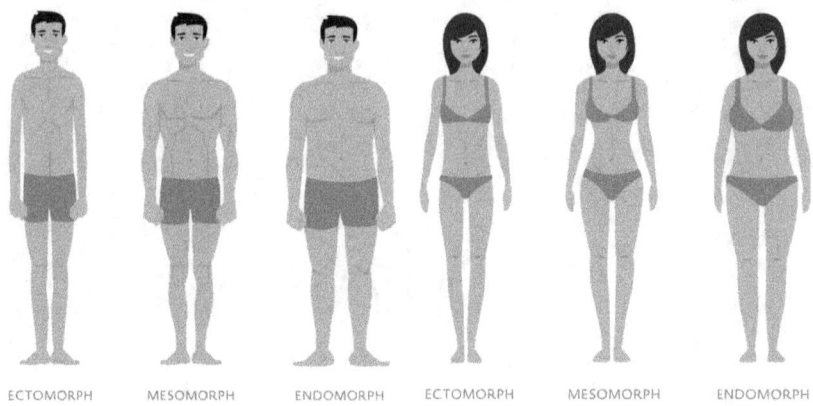

ECTOMORPH

Ectomorphs are lean with long, thin legs and arms, narrow chest and shoulders. Their fast metabolism makes it hard to gain weight and build muscle.

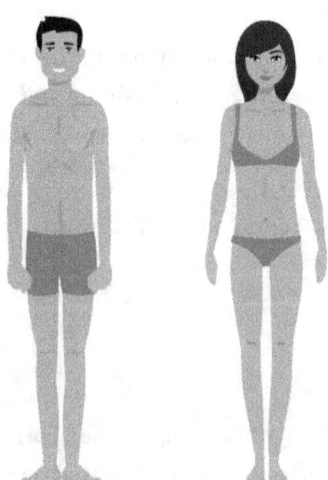

Even if an ectomorph manages to put on weight, they may look slimmer than they are, however they can become remarkably strong and as fit and healthy as someone who looks larger and more muscular.

If this is your body physique and you wish to gain weight and muscles, you'll need to eat like you've never eaten before.

SUGGESTED TRAINING TECHNIQUES FOR ECTOMORPHS

Most ectomorphs' goals are to build lean muscle and put on weight. Ectomorphs tend to eat copious amounts of food but never seem to gain any muscle mass. The type of training I recommend is to begin with very low impact and foundation movements, such as deadlifts, bench squats and military presses.

I suggest a repetition range of 4 to 12, with 4 sets and rest periods in between. Sets should be approximately 60 to 90 seconds and food intake should consist of whole foods and good fats. This will enable ectomorphs to get good results over time. The important thing is steady progress and that weight training does not sacrifice form.

|||||

MESOMORPH

A mesomorph is naturally strong – strong arms and legs, a narrow waist, very little body fat, storing fat evenly across their body, and gains muscle easily.

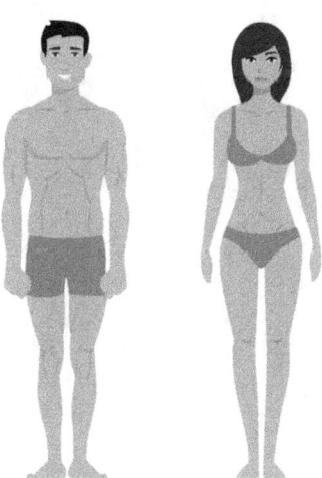

SUGGESTED TRAINING TECHNIQUES FOR MESOMORPHS

A mesomorph body type, in my opinion is the luckiest of the three. They can mix and match their workouts to suit their personal goals. The majority of this body type I have trained have aimed to lose up to about 7 kilos, so I mix it up between high and low volume exercises to see how they personally respond to the workout. Walking and sprinting works, the repetition range should be around 8-15 repetitions, 3 sets and rest periods of around 30 seconds.

Mesomorphs can generally consume more protein but they also need to adhere to proper nutritional principles.

IIIII

ENDOMORPH

The endomorphs have a wider build with a thick ribcage, wide hips, thicker joints and shorter limbs. While they are softer, rounder, curvier, stockier than other physiques, they may have more muscle than either of the other body types. They easily gain fat when adding muscle due to a slower metabolism.

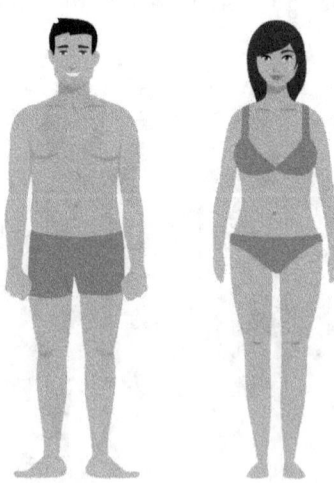

SUGGESTED TRAINING TECHNIQUES FOR ENDOMORPHS

Endomorphs need to be pushed, and pushed hard (controlled of course). They should be doing high repetition ranges from 8–20 reps with reduced rest periods. I would avoid any high impact work initially as this can create injuries. Most endomorphs can have lower limb and knee issues such as shin splints due to the weight they are carrying. They must reduce their calorie intake and put in the extra work in everything they do from nutrition to training to mindset.

|||||

THE IN-BETWEENERS

In-betweeners are a combination of body types i.e. ectomorph/mesomorph or mesomorph/endomorph. In order to optimise your goal, it's important to know which one you are, and train and eat accordingly.

Understanding body type is a big part of the initial process when you get started on the Lean Muscle program.

|||||

FORGET 'DIETING'

It's time to reframe our thoughts. Health and fitness is a priority for a long and fulfilled life and weight loss is simply a side effect of living your healthiest life. Let's kick 'dieting' to the curb and focus on nourishing our body through delicious meals that align with your new lifestyle choice.

Here are a few tips to simplify your diet:
- Eat balanced meals full of unprocessed foods – think grains, protein, vegetables and fruits in a form closest to their natural state.
- Hydrate – it allows your body to work as efficiently as possible.

- Be mindful when restricting your caloric intake – if you fall short on the calories that your body needs to function, your metabolism actually slows down making it harder to lose weight and it can contribute to muscle loss.
- Make movement part of your daily routine – think about what you've eaten and balance it between eliminating extra calories and increasing activity. You can achieve optimum weight, retain muscle in a sustainable routine.

WHAT'S THE DEAL WITH GUT HEALTH?

Gut health has certainly risen to prominence in recent times, there's a buzz word – microbiome – and you may have seen new products appearing in the supermarket such as kombucha, kefir, fermented foods, foods now labelled with prebiotics and/or probiotics. But what does it all mean?

A gut microbiome refers to the community of microorganisms living in your intestines (about 300–500 different species of bacteria in the digestive tract). Many are necessary and incredibly beneficial to a healthy body. A wide variety of good bacteria in your gut can enhance your immune system function, improve symptoms of depression and help combat obesity. Poor gut health has been linked to Crohn's disease, irritable bowel syndrome, non-alcoholic fatty liver disease, obesity and mental health issues.

Dr Elena George, from Deakin's Institute for Physical Activity and Nutrition (IPAN) says, "Gut health is not only determined by what we eat and drink, but also by the amount of physical activity we do, our lifestyle and other environmental factors. But diet and physical activity are interesting because we can all do something about them."[1]

An unhealthy gut may manifest itself through:
- An upset stomach – gas, bloating, constipation, diarrhoea or heartburn.
- Moods, anxiety or depression – the majority of a body's serotonin is produced in the gut; therefore gut damage can impair your ability to sleep well.

- Food intolerances – intolerances to trigger foods can lead to unpleasant symptoms as listed in an upset stomach as well as skin irritations, headaches and autoimmune conditions.
- A high sugar diet – can decrease the amount of good bacteria in your gut and imbalances cause sugar cravings and inflammation.[2]

Dr George says there are two things we can start focusing on to improve our gut: *pre*biotics – feeding the good bugs already in our systems; and *pro*biotics – live bugs that are also good for us, and can be added to our bodies via food or drink or supplements.

The simplest, cheapest, easiest way we can improve our gut health is by eating foods rich in prebiotics – foods rich in fibre that will pass all the way through the digestive system. Foods to steer clear of (except for special occasions) include processed foods, and foods high in salt or sugar.

Fermented foods are rich in probiotics and can be found in things like kombucha, kefir, yoghurt, sauerkraut and pickles.

> *"Always trust your gut. It knows what your head hasn't figured out yet."*
>
> — *Unknown*

YOUR METABOLISM

It pays to understand how the processes in your body work too. Metabolism is the process of converting what we consume, into energy for our body. This physical and chemical process is vital for all of our body's functions: breathing, circulation, repairing cells, moving; everything it does to survive in fact.

The faster your metabolism, the more calories you burn. Factors that affect metabolism include your genetics, age, height, muscle mass and hormonal factors. Research shows that your metabolism slows down with age due to less activity, muscle loss and the aging of your cells and organs.[3]

If we eat more calories than we need, our body will store this excess as fat. It's important to understand that everybody's metabolism works at a different rate, some people are born with a fast metabolism, seeming to eat a lot and not gain weight while some people have slower rates and so are more prone to storing the energy as fat.

METABOLIC SYNDROME

Here is a little extra food for thought to get you off that couch. Metabolic syndrome is the name for a group of conditions that increase your risk of heart disease, stroke and type 2 diabetes. Increased blood pressure, high blood sugar, excess body fat around the waist and abnormal cholesterol or triglyceride levels are all conditions that fall under the definition of metabolic syndrome. More to the point, 35% of Australians have metabolic syndrome and this rate is even higher in people with diabetes.[4]

I know you don't want to become one of the statistics of this condition and hopefully you're starting to reduce your risks by practising the following lifestyle changes:

- Healthy eating – eating balanced meals full of wholegrain and unprocessed foods and reducing your alcohol intake.
- Increasing your physical activity level – at least 30 mins of exercise 5 days a week is recommended.

There is simply no reason not to practise good exercise and a healthy diet.

CAN YOU SPEED UP YOUR METABOLISM TO LOSE WEIGHT?

Yes you can! Extend on the above principles to target and speed up your body's metabolism. Particularly:

- Move your body – the more active you are, the higher your metabolic rate. So take the stairs whenever possible, do your housecleaning with vigour, don't remain stationary for long periods (use a standing desk at work).
- High-intensity workouts (HIIT) are great – HIIT training speeds up your metabolism, even after the workout has finished (known as 'the afterburn').

- Strength training – strength exercises promote the growth of muscle mass and muscle mass increases the number of calories you burn at rest.
- Eat protein – protein increases your metabolic rate by 20-30%.
- Stop starving yourself – when you don't eat enough food, your body reacts by slowing down its metabolic rate, or going into 'starvation mode'. It means even after you stop 'dieting' your body often maintains the same 'slower' metabolic rate, as a survival mechanism.[5]
- Drink more water – hydration leads to an increase in the number of calories burned through water-induced thermogenesis (the production of heat). Drinking cold water has a greater effect, as it requires the body to warm it up to body temperature.
- Get a great night's sleep – inadequate or poor sleep may slow down your metabolic rate, not to mention make you reach for sugar-fuelled foods to 'pick you up'.

FLUCTUATING BODY WEIGHT

Body weight is never stable. It fluctuates depending on food and water intake and exercise. It's crucial to get off the scales and focus on good nutrition and building a healthy mindset. There may be days that you feel driven to raid the fridge, the pantry and everything in between, and then there are days that you feel fulfilled and do not need to consume much food. Remember your bodyweight is determined by the number of calories you consume compared to the number of calories you burn.

I have learnt that as long as I maintain a healthy balanced diet and exercise regime, then the fluctuation really doesn't matter.

The average recommended intake for men is 2500 calories per day and 2000 for women. This can change and shift according to the individual's personal goals. A healthy balance is staying within 5 kg of your ideal body weight.

DON'T BE A SCALE ADDICT

Jumping on the scale will only show your weight without measuring anything else such as muscle mass, fat mass, oxygen, hydration levels etc. There are times the numbers on the scale don't shift, but your shape and your body has changed, so let the mirror and photos be your guide.

Get off the scale and pay attention to how you feel in your clothes and how you look – this is the best indication of success when it comes to weight loss, especially if you are lifting weights, as building muscle will 'gain' weight but not fat.

I strongly recommend taking before pictures and progress pictures along your journey so you can see the changes in your body. If you really want to hop on a scale, there are body composition scales that measure body fat, BMI, muscle and bone mass – most gyms will be able to allow access to this for you.

|||||

WATER – YOUR SECRET WEAPON

Make no mistake water helps your body to exercise efficiently, it provides joints with lubrication and pain relief and decreases your recovery time. It also hydrates your brain, and most importantly promotes weight loss. Drinking cold water contributes to major fat burning if undertaken in an informed, well-planned manner.

Yes, water is such a vital part of the many chemical reactions in the body. If you're going to undertake what this book is all about, i.e. sweating, then you're going to need to increase and monitor your daily water intake.

HOW MUCH WATER SHOULD YOU DRINK?

The amount of water that someone should drink varies greatly from person to person. It depends on how your individual metabolism works, what the temperature is, what you eat, your age and whether you have a medical condition. As a general guideline men should consume between 2.5 to 3.7 litres a day and women between 2 to 2.7 litres a day. Depriving yourself of sufficient water sets your body up to store body fat, as the liver cannot metabolise it into energy as efficiently.

To stay hydrated, it is important to drink *before* you feel thirsty. This is especially important if you are exercising. Drink water regularly throughout the day, not just when you are thirsty.

|||||

SLEEP
YOUR HIDDEN SUPERPOWER

Let's not forgot an easily overlooked factor to maintain good health and energy: sleep. Do you find you prioritise eating well, working out, and drinking lots of fluids, yet your weight loss or fitness regime is not making progress? It's possible you're not getting enough sleep — after all, sleep is just as important for the mind, as for the body. Even if you do everything you can during the day to lead a healthy life, when you suffer from low-quality sleep, it can be difficult to maintain the energy and motivation needed to fulfill your goals to the best of your ability.

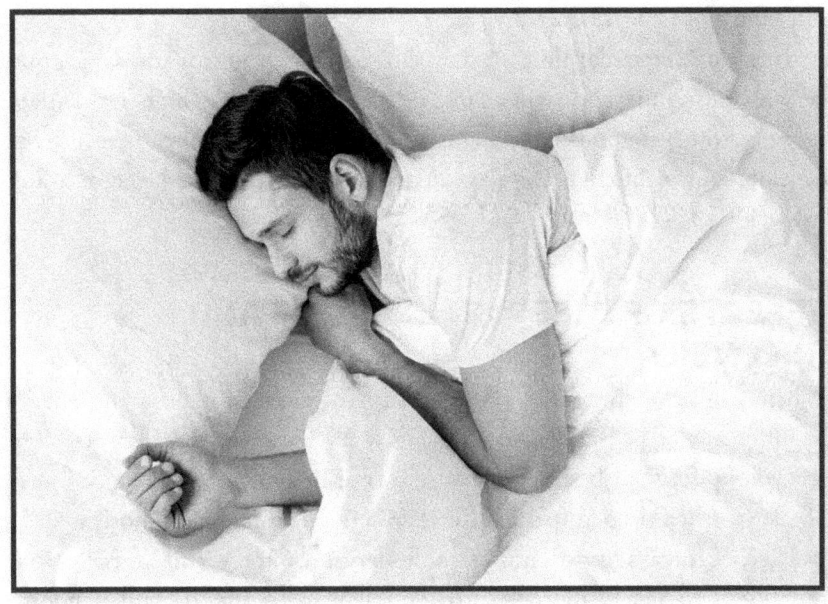

Sleep regulates hormones, boosts brain function, helps with weight management, maintains your immune system, lowers your risk for chronic health conditions and improves athletic performance.

It is recommended healthy adults need between 7-9 hours sleep per night. These figures vary from person to person, and are also dependent on how much exercise you're getting. If you work out often, it's likely you'll need more sleep.

Some of the signs you may *not* be getting enough sleep:
- You don't feel refreshed on waking in the morning.
- When at work you find it difficult to get going in the mornings.
- You are less productive and focused, you forget things or feel fatigued or drowsy throughout the day.
- You're more irritable or moody and lack energy to do things.
- Dark circles under the eyes, dull complexion.
- You wake throughout the night, due to stresses or worries.

SLEEP AND MENTAL HEALTH

Sleep and mental health are closely connected – sleep deprivation affects your psychological state and mental health. Just ask any new parent juggling full time work and a new baby!

There are some alarming studies showing the extent of the association between insomnia and depression, being at a four-fold higher risk than those getting a good night's sleep. [6] Insomnia can also precede the development of bipolar disorder, anxiety, there is even evidence of a link to suicide.[7]

EFFECTS OF SLEEP ON EXERCISE AND RECOVERY

When you are getting the right amount of sleep you have the energy to jump out of bed and move through your day with ease. Proper sleep sets you up for your best performance – your body can deliver quick bursts of energy when needed (perfect for training) and you remain motivated.

Exercise breaks down muscle and depletes energy and muscle from the body. Fatigued muscles provide inadequate support for tendons, ligaments and bones, increasing the risk of strains, sprains, and stress fractures. After exercise your body needs time for hormonal, neurological and structural recovery – tissue repair and muscles, building new structures to make them more fatigue-resistant in the future. Rest and recovery are essential to the success of your training program.

From her studies published in the *Journal of American Medical Association*, researcher Eve Van Cauter says, "We actually know that if we increase deep sleep, we can increase growth hormone,"[8] So more sleep could be just what you need to kick-start your routine to lose body fat or increase muscle!

Lack of sleep influences your body's hormones:
- Leptin inhibits hunger and regulates your food intake and energy expenditure, helping the body to maintain its weight. When leptin decreases with sleep deprivation, it triggers an increase in appetite and food cravings.
- With decreased leptin, your **ghrelin** hormone levels increase thus increasing the feelings of hunger, and your body responds with craving calorie rich foods to compensate for your lack of energy.
- Cortisol controls the body's blood sugar levels and regulates metabolism (among other things). Lack of sleep elevates cortisol levels and increases hunger and may negatively affect your body's metabolism, and affect where your body stores fat – storing more belly fat (visceral adipose tissue 'VAT').[9]
- Sleep deprivation and gut health affect one another cyclically. Even short intervals of sleep deprivation can alter your gut microbiome (remember the 300–500 different species of bacteria in the digestive tract).
- When you restrict calories in a sleep-deprived state your body loses more lean muscle mass than fat (muscle burns more calories than fat), rendering your diet less effective.[10]

Make sleep a priority to give you the energy to live your life to the fullest.

STRIP DOWN

Another surprisingly beneficial tip for a healthy lifestyle is to strip down and sleep naked. For some, this decision is a breeze and science has good news to support the practice. Stripping down may seem like one way to heat things up but scientifically it's all about cooling down.

Sleeping naked:
- Is another way to tell your body it's time to sleep – your body temperature is part of your circadian rhythm for sleep, and can help you fall asleep faster.
- It improves your overall sleep quality when the room temperature is between 15-19C.[11] Too hot or too cold impacts your REM sleep that helps refresh your brain and body.
- Reduces stress and anxiety.[12]
- Helps boost your calorie burning abilities through activating brown fat (a type of fat turned on in cold temps).[13]
- Can lower the risk of heart disease and type 2 diabetes.[14]
- Promotes vaginal health through reducing the risk of a vaginal yeast infection.
- Increases male fertility through keeping testicles at an optimal temperature for sperm health.[15]
- Boosts self-esteem by embracing overall body image.[16]
- Improves your relationship – skin-to-skin contact between adults stimulates the release of oxytocin.[17]

If you aren't comfortable sleeping naked, begin by reducing the number of layers.

|||||

MEN AND TESTOSTERONE

Many of my male clients over 40 continually ask me how I stay strong in my 50s. Firstly we must remember the crucial role testosterone plays in male development such as in the reproductive system and promoting the growth of muscle mass, bone mass and body hair along with the deeper voice testosterone produces over females.

Testosterone also assists in maintaining healthy energy levels and a healthy strong libido. As men age, testosterone slowly decreases at the rate of 1–2% per year for men over the age of 30 and mostly goes unnoticed. In saying this, some men do feel the drop in their testosterone levels, which may contribute to andropause (which is the equivalent to menopause for women – meaning a low testosterone level).

Low levels of testosterone may contribute to loss of muscle mass, reduced body and facial hair, increased breast size, hot flashes, irritability, poor concentration, depression or brittle bones. So if you're not feeling as strong as you should be – that you've lost your mojo – it is important go to a GP who'll take a blood sample to check your testosterone levels and talk about how to regain a healthy balance of hormones again.

You may be asking why I'm mentioning this here. If you find that you're doing all the right things by keeping up with your fitness routine yet still notice an increase in body fat there may be an underlying issue contributing to the lack of muscle growth. I would highly recommend you have a full physical check before embarking on any fitness or high exercise regime. This way, you will be armed with the facts and understand how to move forward.

JUST FOR THE LADIES

Ladies I have not forgotten about you. This book would not be complete without mentioning the many inspiring women I have trained throughout my career, and have been honoured to be a part of their physical and emotional journey, much more than most trainers.

Over the years, I have witnessed the landscape of gyms and training structures completely change. Back in the day, gyms would be filled with alpha males grunting and groaning as they lifted three times their body weight. Nowadays, you can bet your money on walking into a gym and finding that 60% of the people training are women. This is a fantastic turnaround; women now have the freedom to explore their fitness on so many different levels without fear of being judged.

For women, the jump into the world of lifting weights can be daunting. Opinions on ladies and lifting are often inaccurate and stuck in past beliefs from the eras of the '50s and '60s when men and women were culturally assigned to their roles of bread-winner and home-maker. A woman working out back then was a pretty controversial concept as crazy as that sounds today.

As a result of these old myths and assertions about the right training for women, it can be difficult for many women to know how or where to begin. So what better way than to ask Danni, who is living proof of how women and weights combined with a healthy lifestyle is a winning formula.

> **Fred:** How long have you been consistently training for?
> **Danni:** *Since I was 18 years old*
>
> **Fred:** How often do you train?
> **Danni:** *4 times a week incorporating compound movements and isolation*
>
> **Fred:** Do you worry that lifting weights creates a more masculine look?
> **Danni:** *Not at all, the truth is lifting builds muscle and burns fat, quite often the differences in women's physiques come from genetics, how they eat, and the movements, volume, intensity, and load they use in their programming. I find that women need a training regimen that reflects how they want to perform in day-to-day life and what they want to look like.*
>
> **Fred:** Great, do you have any other tips for the ladies reading this book?
> **Danni:** *Yes, set goals for yourself and spend time learning proper technique. Enjoy the process. Be conscious and consistent with your eating habits and correct exercises. Most importantly don't compare yourself to others, and be sure to Sweat Swear Smile regularly!*

Be sure to read the wonderful case studies of some of the inspiring women I have trained in Chapter 7!

IIIII

MY PILOT STUDY

Some time ago now, after listening to some market feedback, I wanted to carefully and constructively delve into the potential of the online space. This meant I would have to test and measure my philosophies to see what could be accomplished in a really focused, intense time period, where people gave it everything for 31 days. Some people had said you can't change your body in that time but I suspected it was possible if the right training tools and support were in place along with a real desire from the client.

I received a truckload of interest in my proposal but in order to test and measure cohesively for my clients and my research, I selected only a few people to take on my 31-Day Pilot Study. Each person came to me with very different goals and different belief systems. However, they all had one key ingredient that made all the difference: desire. Have a look at these case studies that were achieved over only 4 weeks – imagine what you could achieve over 12 weeks!

CASE STUDY: LUKE
TOTAL FAT LOSS 8KG

Luke was 130kg and battling the bulge. He ate mostly the right foods but in the wrong proportions. He was tired often and generally felt unwell. Luke wanted to try and get rid of the stomach and see how muscular he could become in a short amount of time.

Luke's feedback after the four weeks, *"Fred helped me to decrease my portions and my protein intake. He increased cardio and long runs into my program. By the end I felt so much happier in myself. In business you call in the professionals to help you and the same goes for fitness, you seek advice and answers for your journey and Fred is a great mentor, the best wingman you can have by your side to help you conquer your goals."*

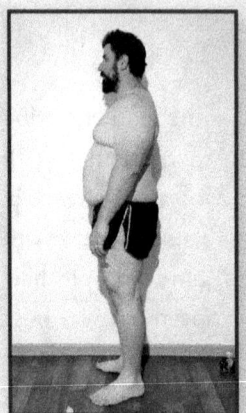
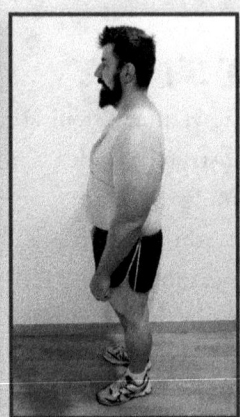

CASE STUDY: JANETTE
TOTAL FAT LOSS 6.5KG, 27.5CM ALL OVER BODY

After having a baby Janette felt challenged to gain motivation, she was recovering from a slipped disc during her pregnancy and lack of sleep made putting exercise and nutrition difficult to prioritise. She would reach for a coffee and something sweet that only gave her a few minutes energy surge. The wrong foods made her feel lazy and unmotivated. She wanted to get back to eating right and exercising regularly, in a short burst of time.

This is what Janette had to say about her experience, *"Week 4 results are in and I am so happy with what I've achieved. Would not have done this without the support of Fred Liberatore, he definitely knows his stuff!"*

Janette didn't really have a target weight loss, she just wanted to feel good again so I was thrilled that after the four weeks Janette felt improved all over and said she had become a better person to herself and her family!

Watch Janette's testimonial at leanmuscle.com.

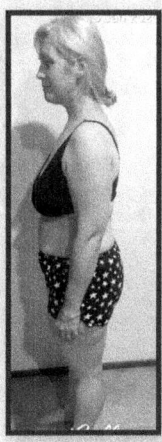
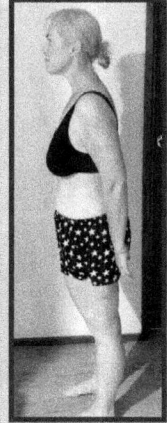
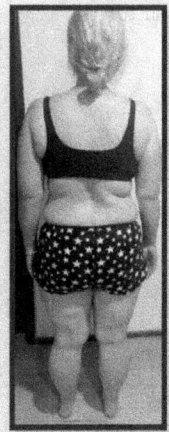
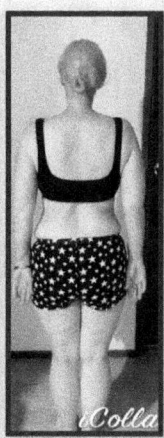

CASE STUDY: CHRIS
TOTAL FAT LOSS 7.2KG

Chris had overindulged in comfort food and alcohol and he was feeling aches and pains in his body for the first time, his self-confidence took a hit. Chris wanted to take better care of himself through nutrition and weight training to recapture his confidence and positivity.

At the end of the month's program Chris said the following, *"It's been a great experience and I'm really happy with my results. A total of 7.2kgs was lost but what you are unable to see is the amount of positivity between my ears; that is where my best work was done. Thanks for the support and opportunity Fred!"*

Chris told me he felt a sense of pride for what he had achieved through his determination and sacrifice and in his words that is, *"One of the most satisfying feelings one can experience."* What an inspiring perspective!

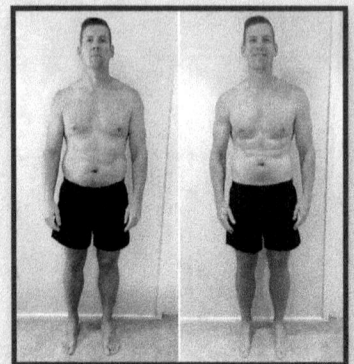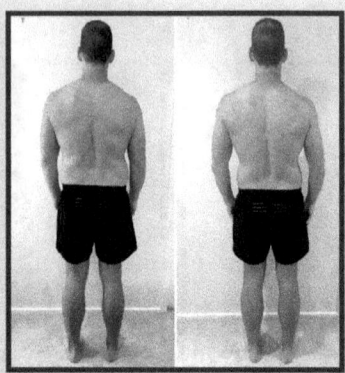

SO HOW WERE THESE RESULTS ACHIEVED?

All the candidates were trained using an online coaching and training program over four weeks. They all received two group-coaching calls a week and had all their questions answered. I used this time to encourage and support them the whole way through. It was a great platform to share their challenges during the week with the group and take on some feedback.

They also looked at the next week's goals and were given detailed videos of exercises with explanations showing them what to move on to next. They also received written material as well as meditation exercises to do and they all felt this is what gave them the edge. They all followed the instructions down to the letter, being very principled in their approach to their personal fitness journey and they all held themselves accountable to the program and to me as their trainer.

These guys really showed the potential for online training and getting those targeted results if you start with a game plan and support from me. Now that you are armed with information about your body before you begin your training, let's look at what you need to know about nutrition in the next chapter.

CHAPTER 4

NUTRITION

Right off the bat I can tell you I'm not a qualified nutritionist. However I have done food coaching in the past and what I am about to tell you has worked with my clients because I did two things well with them – I tested and measured. Let's break down your understanding and relationship with food further by going through some really important nutrition factors.

YOUR RELATIONSHIP WITH FOOD

Everyone comes to me with a different set of beliefs, especially about nutrition. I believe a lot of it stems from your upbringing and your environment. For example, growing up with Italian parents, I couldn't fault the Mediterranean diet, a balanced approach to nutrition. Mum would never reward us with chocolates, carbohydrate or sugar laden foods – they were never in the house, instead when we finished playing sport there would always be fresh fruit on the table.

To this day, the smell of basil takes me back to making homemade tomato sauce amongst the camaraderie of family members helping. Dad would save the 750ml long neck beer bottles and sterilise them. We'd prepare the tomatoes, crushing them and filling the bottles with the homemade sauce and basil. Next they'd be capped and layered in a big 44-gallon drum (with rags or newspapers between the layers) and cooked in the drum, then they would cool in the drum overnight before being stored away. I used to hear some of the bottles explode during the night. Mum would make her famous lasagne and we would finish it off with a nice freshly picked salad from the garden.

When it comes to food, start thinking of it in two components:
1. Recreational – food is a great way to celebrate and get together with friends and family.
2. Nutritional – eating fresh food every day to fuel your body.

The key is understanding how to balance the two aspects and importantly not to overeat, stop before you feel 'full'. We live in a fortunate era and country where food is in abundance and it can be hard to resist the array and the supply of food. However we need to recognise the limit of what our body actually needs.

Sure, you can go on a quest to lose weight, but this doesn't mean you need to deny yourself food that you enjoy. Instead I'm saying know your limits and know when to stop. Once you take control of that, everything changes from there.

For example do you love chocolate but sometimes can't resist eating half the block? Try switching to dark chocolate and limit yourself to two squares and savour the taste. Or you could switch to chocolate with no added sugar and limit yourself to one serve. Start to notice when (and importantly why) you eat the chocolate or whichever processed food and think of strategies to combat the craving (we'll discuss cravings soon) and avoid that situation.

Also be conscious of where you are and why you're there, don't be fixated on the food. True enjoyment comes from the people you're spending time with and the environment.

When my clients come to me with food issues, firstly I find out what their relationship with food is – do they use it as a crutch or a comfort – and adjust things from there. If you can adjust their attitude and relationship with food, then chances are you can adjust the weight, so change what food means to you and you will have a much better experience.

Remember to be kind to yourself in the process. If you obsess about weight loss, you're missing the point and it can be a hollow, unsustainable weight loss without any of the life-changing benefits of changing your *health* and the way you feel about yourself. You're not really achieving what you're capable of. Focus on overall wellbeing, which optimises your whole life.

EVERYDAY NUTRITIONAL FOOD

This is what your diet consists of on a regular basis. It is important you adopt a healthy eating plan incorporating all the essential whole foods your body needs in order to thrive and remain healthy. I believe nutritional foods should be 80% of your daily intake of food. The majority of your food should essentially consist of protein, carbs, fats and foods closest to their natural form. Eating healthy, real food is how your body heals and repairs itself. Keep hydrated of course, with plenty of water throughout the day.

Here is a guide to incorporate healthy foods in your daily diet to boost immunity and help your body heal and repair.
- Berries are one of those foods that have the nutrients your body needs and taste great. Full of antioxidants, they are a treat for those days you are craving something a little sweeter.
- Fish is full of omega-3 fatty acids and protein, which helps in the prevention of heart disease and adds to the essential protein intake needed for healthy and lean muscle.
- Leafy green vegetables are a great source of vitamin A, C and calcium as well as the essential fibre we all need. These are *always* a great addition to your meals.
- Nuts are an excellent way of introducing and including essential plant protein and good fats (monounsaturated), which help in reducing

- the risk of heart disease. Limit these to a handful a day.
- Olive oil is a great source of vitamin E, monounsaturated fats and it tastes amazing either cooked or raw. Olive oil in moderation is one of those versatile ingredients that can be incorporated every day. Choosing olive oil over butter or margarine will help keep your body healthy.
- Whole grains are full of fibre, B vitamins and minerals amongst other great nutrients. Adding whole grains in your diet will help in lowering cholesterol and protect against heart disease. You can include these in your diet through many ways, including oatmeal and breads.
- Yoghurt is a great source of protein, calcium and probiotics; choose only high quality natural yoghurt. Stay away from added fruit yoghurts or flavoured yoghurt as these include added sugars.
- Cruciferous vegetables are an excellent source of fibre, vitamins and nutrients and are thought to help in the prevention of some cancers. These vegetables include broccoli, brussels sprouts, cabbage, kale, cauliflower, radishes, turnips and many more.
- Legumes cover a wide range of foods which are all a great source of fibre, they are a plant based protein and folate rich. Legumes include adzuki beans, Anasazi beans, black beans, black-eyed peas, fava beans, garbanzo beans (chickpeas), kidney beans, lentils, lima beans, pinto beans and split peas.
- Tomatoes are high in vitamin C and can be included in your diet, raw or cooked. They are an easy and versatile ingredient to add to any dish.

RECREATIONAL FOODS

This is the remaining 20% of your nutritional intake of food. This is the food that you consume on an occasional basis i.e. family dinners, outings, parties etc. It is okay to have a little bit extra, as long as you are consistent with the 80% previously discussed. Growing up on a Mediterranean diet, I was taught wholesome, healthy food was important. We made our own pasta sauce and pasta from scratch; you get the idea. We never ate foods full of preservatives, junk food or processed foods.

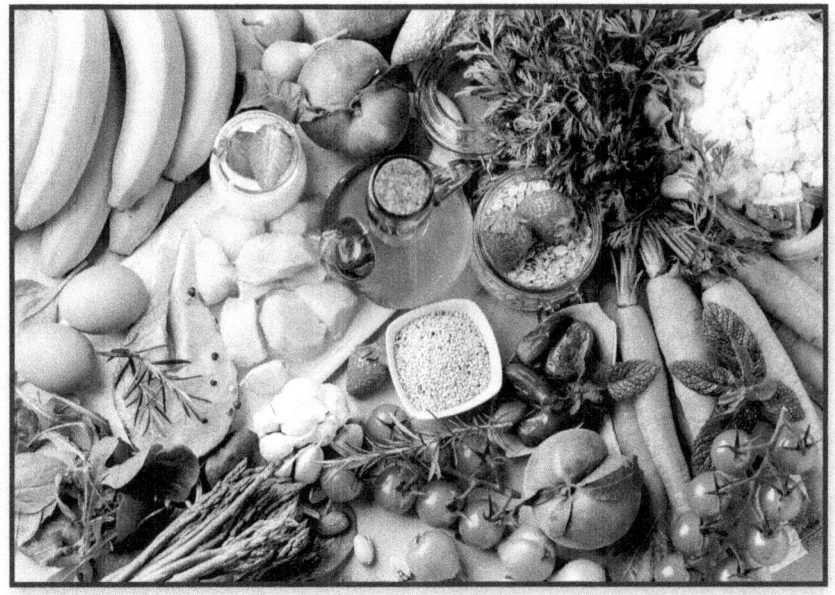

When you sign up to my 12-Week Challenge at leanmuscle.com, you will instantly receive a copy of my 100+ page nutritional book to arm you with knowledge to get started and keep you heading in the right direction. Included in this book is information about carbohydrates, proteins, glycaemic index chart and so much more.

DON'T OVEREAT OR UNDER-EAT

Surprisingly, many people become so caught up in what are they are doing, they neglect to eat properly throughout the day (under-eating) while at the other end of the scale are those that tend to overeat in one sitting. A good rule of thumb is never go hungry but never eat until you are full either.

Eat until you are satisfied and stop before it becomes that full, bloated feeling. And never go hungry to the point where you feel hunger pangs (with the exception of an intermittent fast which I will talk about later).

It is a balancing act but you soon recognise what suits your needs. When building muscle, smaller more frequent meals throughout the day are beneficial, providing a steady supply of protein. I generally space meals between three and four hours, so I'll often have six small meals a day. Keeping your blood sugar levels in check is important to maximise fat burning, another good reason behind eating small, frequent meals.

Understanding your genetic predisposition and body type will help you balance your intake with the right amount of 'fuel' to stoke your fire! Sometimes it comes down to using the food scales to keep a tight reign but generally you'll come to recognise by sight what portions suit your needs.

CRAVINGS

Everybody has cravings: for some it's sugar, others carbs, some a little of everything. Usually when people crave food, the food is high in sugar and fats and this is a no-go zone on a fitness and healthy eating plan. Cravings are caused when there is an imbalance of the hormones leptin and serotonin, which is responsible for pleasure, reward and memory. A great way to combat cravings is to make sure you are having full, nourishing-rich foods in your meals and healthy snacks during the day. You want to make sure you are drinking lots of water too.

If you feel that the cravings occur more often, a good strategy is to write about your craving or what is happening in your life at that moment. Then reconfirm your goals and look at what is important for you, and keep busy away from the temptation. This is a great way to refocus and understand if the craving is emotional or physical. Think about how you will feel after you've eaten the craving, it is often enough to deter you. Part of any big journey requires healing and letting go of old patterns and disruptive behaviours. Learn to listen to your body and understand what it is telling you.

HOW TO HANDLE CRAVINGS

Cravings can take control of your thoughts and when you succumb to cravings that aren't beneficial to your goals, they make losing weight nearly impossible.

How do you curb those intense cravings? By eating foods that will stabilise your blood sugar, delivering a steady flow of energy to your brain and muscles such as:

- Protein rich foods like eggs, lean cuts of free-range chicken or grass-fed meat, fatty wild-caught fish such as salmon or prawns.
- Fibre rich foods such as oatmeal, sprouted-grain breads and pastas, bran, barley, and quinoa.
- Vegetables and fruit such as broccoli, broccoli sprouts, pumpkin and pumpkin seeds, okra, kale, avocados, berries.
- Dairy such as kefir, yoghurt and cheeses.
- Herbs and spices that stabilise sugar cravings: black pepper, cardamon, cayenne pepper, cumin, fenugreek, ginger, ginseng, oregano, turmeric, cinnamon, cloves, nutmeg etc.
- Nuts, nut butters and flax seeds.

Avoid food high in sugar and processed foods. Combine high glycaemic foods with fat or protein to slow the rate of digestion and to better balance your blood sugar.

Interested to know more? Email me at info@leanmuscle.com with the subject line 'reference guide'.

CHEAT MEALS

I think a cheat meal is fine and serves a purpose, however try not to turn it into a cheat day! That is harder to recover from and can demotivate you.

Why am I okay with cheat meals? Research has shown that a cheat meal can be important to your diet as a way to regulate hormones. Leptin regulates your appetite and controls satiety, and ghrelin tells you when you're hungry. When you follow a lower calorie diet to lose weight your ghrelin levels can increase.

Over time your body will grow used to a low-calorie diet, it will adjust accordingly and can plateau. A cheat meal high in calories and carbohydrates can assist in jumpstarting your metabolism, regulating these hormones by encouraging the body to keep burning these calories, instead of adjusting to this lower intake.[1]

A cheat meal can be the reward at the end of the weekly tunnel and can help you stay more motivated to remain healthy 80% of the time.

If you choose the best quality ingredients, a cheat meal can look something like this:
- Love a burger? Choose all natural, grass-fed, hormone-free red meat.
- Prefer pizza? Make the dough from scratch so you know what ingredients you're consuming.
- Craving a cookie? Use almond meal or coconut flour instead of wheat flour and coconut sugar or monk fruit sweetener instead of sugar.

Remember there are always healthier substitutions. Try and resist the garlic bread and soda ☺. Not a fan of cooking? Go for fresh ready-made meals with as few ingredients as possible.

Try and plan ahead, don't go overboard and if you have to have a cheat meal, be smart about it. Remember food is fuel for the body. Consuming large amounts of calories in one sitting will leave you with low energy levels making you feel sluggish and tired. It's important you remain vigilant to avoid getting carried away and losing control.

WIN THE NIGHTLY BATTLE

During the day the body is (usually) continually active as we move about, but after the evening meal most people sit down to watch TV or spend time on their device or read a book, thus shifting their body to inactivity.

Although your metabolism does not slow at night, it isn't releasing as many hormones as during the day, so you need to be careful of the types of food you put into your body at night.

I recommend the evening meal to be the last of all carbohydrates for the day. Since eating carbs increases glycogen levels, it is important to limit carb intake at night if you're looking to burn fat. Keep them low so when you wake up in the morning that fat-burning can resume.

If you are hungry and need to eat every two hours, stick to other macronutrients such as protein and healthy fats: cottage cheese, almonds, a tablespoon of peanut butter or coconut oil etc. Cottage cheese is best because it contains casein protein, a slower digesting protein that will keep your muscles supplied with protein throughout the night. Cottage cheese also has an extremely high biological value (around 85%), which is ideal for muscle growth. It is also high in calcium helping to increase bone strength and density, essential in fighting off osteoporosis.

INSIDE OUT

Did you know that the natural state of the human body is slightly alkaline? Your blood must maintain a slightly alkaline pH of 7.30 to 7.45.

However, today's lifestyle is causing our bodies to accumulate acid waste, which creates a potential breeding ground for all kinds of modern diseases. We eat more foods now that are low in energy such as biscuits and cakes and this excess acid waste causes our natural waste disposal systems (kidney and liver) to be completely overloaded.

In response, our body's homeostasis (automatic balancing system) stores the acid waste in fatty deposits. Just as acid on metal creates rust, similarly acid waste in the body oxidises and ages the body.

Your body's pH balance is referred to as its acid-base balance; it is the levels of acids and basis in your blood at which your body functions best.

Acidic and basic are two extremes that describe chemicals, just like hot and cold are two extremes that describe temperature. Mixing acids and bases can cancel out their extreme effects, much like mixing hot and cold water can even out the water temperature.

Signs of imbalance can be:
- Low energy, fatigue, chronic fatigue
- Sugar cravings, caffeine cravings
- Poor digestion, excess weight
- Unclear thinking
- Dehydrated skin
- Joint pain, arthritis
- Candida

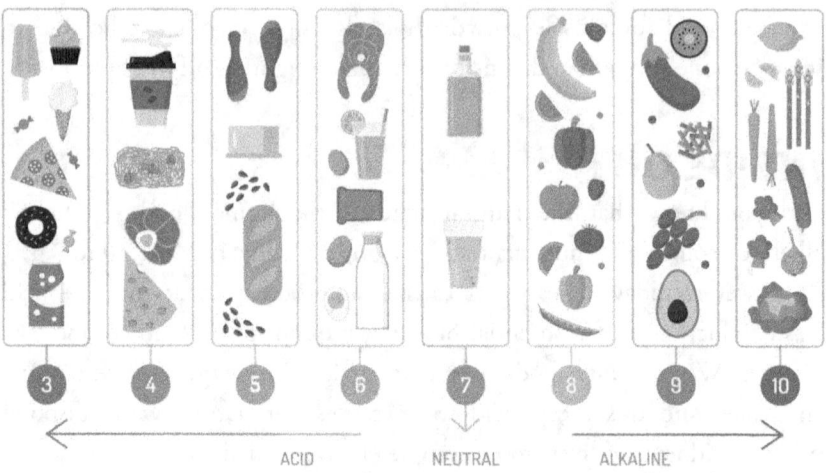

Alkalise whenever you get the chance by consuming:
- Vegetables: asparagus, watercress, parsley, broccoli, spinach, celery, chlorella, collard greens, kale, spirulina, barley grass, wheat grass, wild greens etc.
- Protein: tofu, eggs, whey protein powder, cottage cheese, chicken breast, almonds and brazil nuts.
- Fruit: apples, apricots, cherries, berries (except blueberries), grapes, kiwis, melons (all varieties), mangoes, passion fruit, dates, figs, pears etc.
- Alkaline water: drink water with a pH between 7–10.

YOUR BODY IS A STORAGE UNIT

Every time you put something in your body, you need to think of it as putting food in a storage unit, a *small* storage unit. If your body gets filled with too much food, you have a disaster: an overweight, obese mess with no muscular definition because it is covered in adipose tissue 'storing' energy in the form of fat (storing it for a rainy day in biological terms).

Every time you put something into your body, you need to make sure you expend that energy. The food you ingest should either be going towards muscle repair or producing energy to get you through your workouts. This practice is part of the preparation of knowing your calories in and out, not religiously, but a sensible lifestyle adjustment.

I don't want you over-training either; this will create an improper hormonal environment for muscle building and fat burning. It's all a balancing act that needs to be followed properly but that's what I'm here for.

CUT OUT THE JUNK

Junk food is exactly that; junk to your body – it's highly processed, made of high sugar, or carbs converting to sugar or high in the wrong type of fat. It contains empty calories with no nutritional value. These foods typically go straight to your body fat stores and instead of an energy high, you feel lethargic and unmotivated.

Eliminate all processed foods and replace them with natural whole foods. Be aware of ingredients added to foods to enhance flavours such as MSG and hydrogenated oils that extend shelf life. You'll find out more as part of the 12-Week Challenge in the included nutrition ebook.

12-DAY CLEANSE

The decision to kick start your fitness may be triggered by a desire to lose weight, tone up or in response to symptoms of sluggishness, lacking energy, recurrent infections or difficulty coping with stress. Following a health and fitness plan helps to rid the body of potentially harmful chemicals, as well as improving the function of important elimination organs such as the liver, kidneys, intestinal tract and skin.

I suggest beginning with a 12 day cleanse. This helps to remove toxins from your body and will soon help you feel more energised. You can expect to experience headaches and fatigue due to the body withdrawing from caffeine and sugar. Generally, you start to feel better by Day 5. Here is a guide to a 12-day cleanse.

What to eliminate:
- Alcohol
- Coffee
- Sugar
- Fried foods
- Bread, cereals, pasta, cakes and biscuits
- Soft drink/soda i.e. coke and diet coke
- Starchy vegetables – potato, parsnip, pumpkin and corn
- Fruit juice

What to include:
- Unlimited vegetables especially the greens
- Lean meats such as chicken or fish
- Sweet potato
- Green tea
- Fresh vegetable juice
- Cheese – 50g cottage, feta or ricotta
- Roasted chickpeas
- Limit fruit to 1 serve of low G.I. fruit – all berries, apples, pears

Daily exercise:
- Moderate aerobic exercise for at least 45 minutes every day to keep the released toxins moving. Low impact is best.

Hydration:
- Drink at least 2–4 litres of water per day.
- Drinking water before a meal takes the edge off the appetite.
- Water ensures normal bowel and kidney function to rid the body of wastes as well as stored fat.
- Drinking water alleviates fluid retention, since only when the body gets plenty of water will it release the stored water.

This easy recipe is an example of the many practical recipes I will provide you with along your 12-Week Challenge. It's a great one to incorporate into a 12-day cleanse.

RECIPE | TUNA AND COTTAGE CHEESE DIP

Servings: 1

INGREDIENTS

- 125g springwater tuna
- 60g cottage cheese
- 1 tbsp. mayonnaise
- 1 tbsp. balsamic vinegar
- 1 tspn. UDO's oil blend
- Salt and pepper to taste
- Vegetable sticks: carrots, celery, cucumber, broccoli

METHOD

1. Strain tuna. In a mixing bowl, combine the tuna, cheese, mayonnaise, vinegar and oil.
2. Season if desired. Mix until thoroughly combined. Serve with vegetable sticks.

What a simple healthy, homemade snack at any hour. Enjoy!

ALCOHOL

Excessive drinking has negative impacts on your fitness and body full stop. Understanding what alcohol does to your body can help you avoid undoing all of your great work. Drinking in moderation is commonly considered to be one alcoholic drink for women per day and two drinks for men. However there is no 'moderation' if you're trying to lose weight because alcohol is an *extra calorie* – the body can't process or utilise it for energy so it adds on weight; it's counterproductive.

Alcohol affects hydration. Alcohol is a diuretic and speeds up the loss of water and electrolytes needed for proper hydration. If you are dehydrated before you start working out, your performance isn't going to be as good.

Alcohol is a sedative, impairing reaction time, balance and hand-eye coordination. You're unable to perform at your highest level. Alcohol is a toxin to the body. Once consumed, your body works to remove it from its system. Your liver works harder and has an effect on your metabolism.

Drinking multiple drinks in the evening affects REM sleep, impacting the immune system and impairing protein synthesis for muscle development and maintenance. A 2014 study, where athletes knocked back a few drinks after an intense workout showed their muscle building and recovery, also known as protein synthesis, decreased by 37%.[2] Drinking interferes with your ability to grow and maintain muscle.

When it comes to muscle recovery, it extends recovery time with your liver metabolising the alcohol in your system and engaging the kidneys and digestive system. My recommendation is to stop drinking altogether until you reach your goal, then when you are out socially and would like a drink, drink in moderation.

EATING OUT

Dining out should be a joyful experience, you're working hard and you want to give yourself a reward and besides, we already talked about the 80/20 rule whereby food is seen as nutritional *and* recreational. So here is the recreational component with a few tips I have put together for eating out.

1. Do your research: jump online and check out the menu of the restaurant. If the menus aren't online, give them a call to see if they can cater for you. You want to avoid deep fried foods and sauces, and keep the experience a pleasurable one.
2. For goodness sake do not load up on carbs, aka the 'free' bread basket. Resist the temptation by saying, "No thanks," and have the waiter take the basket with them – out of sight is out of mind!

3. Choose either an entrée or a dessert but not both, so you don't leave the restaurant feeling like you've swallowed a truck tyre. Don't eat with your eyes so only choose one extra course with your main meal if you really want to.
4. I love any type of fish, so why not have a fish dish at the restaurant and load up on a green salad and green veggies – you can't go wrong.
5. If you're going to have a dessert, why not divide it up with others in your party? Often you only need a few tastes to feel rewarded and recognise a good limit.

Whatever you decide though, absolutely enjoy it and ditch the guilt. Good food is an important part of life, family and friends.

SHOPPING ONLINE OR INSTORE

By now, this book should be piquing your interest in how to really clean up your diet. As we've mentioned, depriving yourself of your favourite foods can set you up for failure when you give in to the temptation and binge. So how do you avoid blowing all your good work?

Preparation is the key to your success however you shop. Firstly stop dropping into the supermarket on your way home from work when you're more likely to succumb to grabbing something quick because you're low on energy or are feeling hungry. Go shopping after you've eaten and you'll shop far more sensibly using foresight for the coming week.

If you arrive home late and tired, complacency will naturally creep in unless you are prepared for this scenario. So it's really important to prepare meals before you need them. Weekends are a great time to prepare your meals for the coming week. I recommend:

Planning your meals for the week ahead of time and write your grocery list in detail.

Shop for everything at once either:
- In store – the ideal time to shop is after a meal when your appetite is satiated and strong enough to avoid temptation and you're more likely to stick to your list.

- Online – perfect if you succumb easily to temptation. Shopping online is a timesaver. If you haven't shopped online from your local supermarket in the past, the first time will take longer as you set up lists and populate them with foods you purchase every week from different sections but then every order afterwards your list will be saved ready to tweak for the next order.

Once you arrive home or your order is delivered, unpack your groceries and prepare them ready to use e.g. wash your lettuce and store it in an airtight container. You'll be more likely to make a quick salad if it's half ready anyway.

Allocate some time to prepare your meals for the week – lunches and snacks especially. Cook that roast and shred the meat ready for lunch wraps, tacos etc.

INTERMITTMENT FASTING

Not only have I experienced the benefits of intermittent fasting, my clients have tried, tested and measured the results with excellent outcomes. From my experience fasting is a great approach to learn about and include into your routine when commencing a fitness plan.

It is about including a new behaviour which will not only benefit you in the long run, adding more energy and stamina but fasting will help you with your weight loss goals. There is a lot of science and research behind this method that shows intermittent fasting rejuvenates the body at a cellular level and has been used for centuries around the world with excellent results.

Intermittent fasting is where you cycle between periods of eating and voluntary fasting. There are different methods of intermittent fasting – alternate day fasting, periodic fasting and time-restricted fasting (e.g. the most popular 16/8 method, the eat-stop-eat 24-hour method or the 5:2 diet). People already 'fast' every day while they sleep. Intermittent fasting is as simple as extending that fast a little longer. Fasting exists in various religious practices e.g. Christianity, Hinduism, Islam, Jainism and Buddhism.

I stumbled across fasting many years ago with a client who was fasting for religious reasons. This piqued my interest so I decided to try it out for myself and failed miserably. When I came out of the fasting, I ate everything in sight, seriously! But that didn't stop me, I wanted to know more, so I decided to do my own research on the matter.

I came across a book called *Eat Stop Start* by Brad Pilon. After that it all became clear, technically it's 24 hours but you are not going an entire day without food. So I tried again and although I kept looking at the clock to see when I could eat, when the time came something marvellous happened, I didn't gorge myself, I felt disciplined.

I decided once a week I would simply fast without making a big deal about it, and to this day I still practise 24-hour fasting. I believe it gave me a whole new way of looking at the way the body works, energetically I felt brand new, and it was insane! There is an initial withdrawal that happens (caffeine and sugar) but when you persist, there is elation and energy. I have found fasting strengthens your relationship with food and I highly recommend fasting, the right way.

After a new client's initial assessment I recommend fasting once a week to once a fortnight. As usual, always discuss this with your GP or other health professional before taking on a huge change. When I work with clients, I come up with the right nutritional practice for them, show them how to fast correctly and support them every step of the way.

What you need to know for now is to pick a day and time to fast and choose your favourite tea or mineral water and an organic bone broth. Through testing I have found beginning anywhere from 12:30–2:00pm for a 24-hour period is optimal, as you never go a full day without eating i.e. 12:30pm Saturday to 12:30pm Sunday. And when you begin introducing food, start with clean food such as protein, vegetables, salads and fruit etc.

Take a look at my fasting video at leanmuscle.com.

|||||

SUPPLEMENTS

Using supplements is a personal choice rather than a requirement. I have added grass-fed protein to my nutrition plan since getting into fitness. Often people use supplements as a crutch, rather than as the word defines – a supplement to be used in conjunction with hard work, determination, diligence, and good nutrition.

While a lot of supplements can be beneficial, some can be extremely dangerous, so it's important for you to be careful of what you put into your body. I suggest you speak with your health professional before taking anything you are unsure of. Remember everything requires balance.

CAFFEINE

Be extra careful of any stimulants like caffeine before workouts. A little can help with your exercise regime however, too much can lead to desensitisation and therefore have an adverse effect.

VITAMINS AND MINERALS

Vitamins and minerals such as iron, calcium and vitamin C are essential nutrients the body needs in small amounts to function at optimal levels. These are all found in lean proteins and leafy green vegetables. Create and maintain a healthy and balanced diet and you will reduce the need for the extra supplemental support.

PROTEIN

Having a protein supplement is okay, however eating as close to nature as possible will give you the best outcome and your body will thank you for it. There is nothing wrong with having a scoop of protein powder for the days you are short on time, go for natural and grass-fed to support your needs and health in the best possible way.

Doing your research will help immensely in choosing the right one for you. If you want to increase your lean muscle growth, be sure to choose a protein powder with a high biological value (how well the body absorbs and uses the protein). Whey protein and isolates are very good too.

Like most manufactured foods, protein powders are not all created equal. It is so important you choose one that is *not* denatured (processed and altered) and is free from any chemicals or additives. Do not get sucked in by the marketing and always look at the ingredients list and nutritional facts. If you do not recognise all the ingredients, then it's definitely a no-go. If you recognise the ingredients and it makes sense, if it's low in sugar and free from fillers, then you have a winner. Education is key in everything and it's important you take responsibility for what you are putting in your body.

FOCUS ON THE NOW AND NOT AN ALL OR NOTHING APPROACH

Does this sound familiar? You start a weight loss or exercise plan then veer off course, and having already blown it decide you might as well continue being bad and start over again the next day or next Monday?

Well I want you to stop and think differently! Firstly, let's drop the word 'diet' from your vocabulary. We've grown up with the term diet bandied around as a short term eating habit that's restricted to dropping weight quickly.

Instead let's change it to a lifestyle choice, where our 'why' and short or long-term goals guide our way. Make your goals realistic and chunk them down into smaller goals that are attainable and help you chart your progress. It's easy to get derailed when our end game is a long way away.

Short and mid term goals help you focus on the here and now, keep you motivated and focused on your decisions about food and exercise, then drill down to daily tasks to help you move forward.

TIPS FOR SUCCESS

1. Set a goal that excites and scares you at the same time – if your goal doesn't excite you, it's too small and you remain in your comfort zone.
2. Align your values with your goals – when they're congruent, it's easier to say no to that which derails your efforts.
3. Do the math – a lean body comes from decreasing the calories consumed by changing the fuel type and increasing the calories burned.
4. Be consistent – results are achieved when you consistently work at it every day.
5. Be the captain of your own ship – there are going to be internal storms in the disguise of self-doubt. If you cannot weather the storms, you'll never reach new shores.
6. Use your failures – use each learning as your motivational rocket fuel. When you 'failed', what did you learn, what can you change to create a different result?
7. Get a personal trainer – support, encouragement and accountability will make all the difference in moving past doubts and achieving new heights.

CHAPTER 5

EXERCISES

TRAIN BAREFOOT

Time to let you in on one of my best-kept secrets. Being completely grounded is key to your movements, especially when working with weights. The energy you send through your entire body begins at your feet; they are your foundation. When you're grounded, you're present in the moment and in complete control of your mental and emotional self. The secret is training barefoot, yes, barefoot! For everything – warm up, cool down, strength and conditioning training, weight lifting, everything!

Why is that, I hear you ask. There are 26 bones, 33 joints, over 100 ligaments and approximately 7,800 nerves in each foot. Their complexity allows the body to walk, run and climb all while balancing the weight of the body in response to change. Every foot movement impacts your whole body.

Sensory input is heightened with skin contact to the surface you're standing on. It allows the position of your joints and the tension of your muscles to be finely calculated each moment. When you put on socks and shoes you lose a significant amount of input – you can't sense the ground beneath you and so some muscles shut off because they rely on the support of the shoe which affects your entire movement pattern, influences your lift and the amount of force you are able to exert.[1]

Training barefoot not only improves the strength and mobility of your feet but also your proprioception. This means sensing the position and movement of your body and responding accordingly. Try this activity to see what I mean: using bare feet, stand on one foot with the other foot in front of it, now close your eyes. Do you feel steady? If not, your proprioception needs some development.

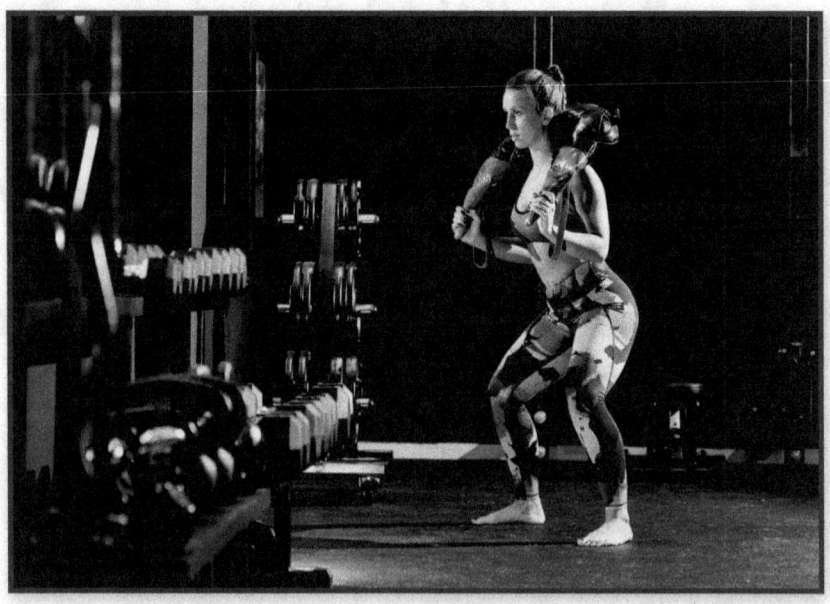

Barefoot is the foundation all movement comes from; otherwise your body will activate other muscles to compensate for the lack of sensation coming from your feet. This can result in imbalances, improper muscle use and poor joint alignment. All body parts work in unison and compromising your footing can negatively affect other parts of your body.

I know what you're thinking, "Okay Fred, that sounds great but what if my gym won't allow me to train barefoot?"

Honestly, I suggest changing gyms — most owner-operated gyms understand the principle and advantage of barefoot training. "What if I drop a weight on my foot Fred?" If you are barefoot and grounded, it's unlikely you'll drop a weight. You wouldn't be reaching that weight and level of training without serious practice.

TRAINING OPTIONS

Having a good personal trainer is like having a good accountant; you can rely on them to manage the workload, keep you up-to-date and help you grow when you're ready by throwing challenges at you. A good personal trainer is proactive (not reactive) and can see the issue arriving well before you think of it, and provides you with an executable plan of attack.

Having a personal trainer does one major kick-arse thing above all others; it keeps you accountable. Heck, even I have a personal trainer because it's a great way to check in and also get my arse kicked if I'm not keeping my end of the agreement.

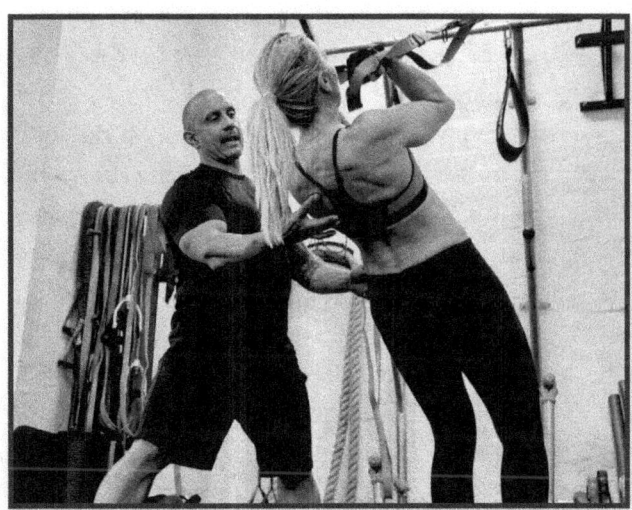

The relationship can be short, medium or long term. A good trainer never holds back, constantly testing and measuring their student and vice versa. For some, the 12-week journey may be enough to create momentum, others see it as part of their daily ritual. Whatever you decide, be sure to hold on to a great trainer, as they are often hard to find!

Good personal trainers are fairly booked up during peak times and prices for one-to-one training can be expensive, but don't let that hinder you! Ask about sharing the costs with fellow gym goers and enter the semi private training model where trainers create dynamic and fun workouts that emphasise camaraderie, accountability, motivation and teamwork, a unique experience in which clients thrive.

Semi-private training is more affordable while still giving you access to a personal trainer. I suggest choosing a trainer whose maximum group size is 6 participants to keep it personalised. Larger group classes are often confined to a cookie cutter program. Be sure to try a few different styles of classes and/or trainers to work out what is best for you.

There is a growing trend of online fitness training. Be sure to ask about their qualifications as discussed earlier, otherwise they are just keyboard warriors with no certifications. When done properly, the benefits of an online PT guided program vastly outweighs the disadvantages. Benefits include cost effectiveness (especially if you want to train more than once a week), trackable results, working out at a time that works best for you, exercises designed to be done at home and having a group to connect with for support.

Online trainers like myself provide custom exercise videos with clearly voiced instructions on how to do a specific exercise that you can watch over and over again, and if all else fails, you can always message them with your questions. You have support and fitness advice around the clock and conveniently in your pocket.

Training on your volition is always an option but it's not for the faint hearted. The majority of people need that dedicated person or tribe of people to connect to and feed off their energy. It's so easy to go off track and give up if someone besides yourself doesn't hold you to account.

EXERCISE MYTHS EXPOSED

I've heard every myth there is over my career and I hope I can clear up any myths you might still have with the information here.

1. **No pain no gain.**

This myth is now busted! You do not have to be in pain to gain a great body. Yes, there may be sore muscles the next day, but 'pain' is extreme. If you feel that there is too much pain, you may have caused an injury so I would strongly suggest you go and get this checked by your GP as soon as possible. Never leave an injury untreated for too long.

2. **Machines beat free weights.**

Once again, it is about form and technique, not equipment. You can work out using your own body weight and still form beautifully sculpted muscles.

3. **Resistance training will make me big and bulky.**

Resistance training builds strength and muscles – not necessarily big and bulky.

4. **I do not want to look like a bodybuilder.**

You don't have to look like a bodybuilder to be strong and increase strength, stability and fitness. It's all about what goals you have and tailoring the workout to suit them.

5. **Sit-ups burn belly fat.**

Belly fat is one of the more difficult zones to target. Many people believe that sit-ups will reduce and burn the fat around their belly and abdomen alone. Unfortunately, you cannot focus solely on one aspect of the body and expect that to be reduced. There is no such thing as spot reduction without surgery.

Sit-ups are great at toning, sculpting and strengthening the core muscles of the abdomen, but will not reduce the fat sitting on top of them. Reduction of fat only occurs when you combine exercise and a healthy eating plan.

6. **I should only do intense exercise 30 minutes once a week.**
Say what! You really should be exercising at least 30 minutes a day as well as high intensity workouts up to three times a week or more depending on your personal fitness goals.

7. **Carbohydrates make me fat.**
There is a great misconception about carbs. The truth of the matter is that consuming a large quantity of calories is what makes a person put on weight, not necessarily foods rich in carbs. Carbohydrates are the body's preferred source of fuel for most activities and if you are not eating enough carbs, your body will not be performing at its optimal level therefore your fitness and weight loss goals will be affected as a result.

The trick I have learned over the years is not to completely take carbs out of the diet, but instead change the 'bad' carbs for 'good' carbs. There is such a thing as a healthy carb source such as fruit and vegetables, nuts and seeds, whole grains, beans and legumes to mention a few.

'Good carbs' will also assist in your weight loss journey as they help keep you fuller for longer. These foods also support muscle growth and are a great resource to rely on when embarking on the fitness journey.

I would suggest reducing or eliminating any refined and starchy carbs including white rice, white pasta, processed snacks and sweets. From personal experience, eating some form of healthy carbohydrate straight after a workout (no matter what time) will help restore the depletion of glycogen in the body and keep you sane! Failure to do this will result in your muscles putting the brakes on recovery. So a great way to reward yourself after a fantastic workout would be to consume a bowl of porridge with added protein.

8. Sweating means you're not in shape.

This is a great myth to bust and quite the opposite is true. This book is called *Sweat Swear Smile*! Having these three things as part of your workout goals will help you maintain a healthy attitude and allow you to reach your goals faster.

I really love seeing my clients dripping in sweat after a great workout as it means they have worked really hard and pushed themselves to the limit. As mentioned in the 'Sweating' section of Chapter 1, sweating is the body's natural cooling down mechanism and actually a great thing.

It's really important you rehydrate after a big session in order to replenish what you have lost through sweat. If you are not working hard enough to increase your core temperature, your body will not need to cool down therefore you will not sweat. If you feel that you have worked out really hard and you still aren't sweating, consult your GP and get a full health check to check it out.

9. You shouldn't work out on an empty stomach.

While working out on an empty stomach has its supporters, it's not generally a good idea. It can burn valuable energy that you need for other daily activities such as the concentration needed for working or driving and for moving comfortably through your day.

Exercising on an empty stomach can result in reduced stamina and a drop in blood sugar levels, which can make you feel light headed. You should see your GP if you experience frequent light-headedness. Eat a piece of fruit before your workout to fuel up and remember working up a sweat is a great way to kick off your day. As always, remain hydrated before, during and after your workout.

10. Lifting weights will bulk me up.

Weight lifting is often in the spotlight as people gape at the huge sculpted muscles of bodybuilders. Often people don't realise how bodybuilders must follow a *very* regimented exercise and nutrition plan to design their body. It doesn't just happen by lifting weights.

Individuals increasing muscle mass and decreasing body fat are following a very specific exercise and nutrition program. And ladies, you won't bulk up by accident because your body doesn't produce testosterone at the levels men's bodies produce testosterone (16 times the level of women).

Lifting weights increases strength in your tendons and ligaments, increases bone density (decreased risk of osteoporosis), increases your resting metabolic rate and increases muscle mass (more efficient fat burning). Weights give you a chance to get out of your comfort zone, however it's important to use weights that work for your fitness level to avoid any injuries.

11. Your muscle will turn into fat if you stop working out.
When you exercise, your existing muscles grow larger and stronger, the number of capillaries increases and muscles develop more mitochondria resulting in more defined muscle mass, rather than newly created muscle tissue.

When you decrease the physical activity in your body, your muscles decrease in mass. The increased blood flow required to fuel your cells during exercise is no longer required, your body begins to contract, reducing the size of the capillaries, and the muscle mass decreases.

If your diet provides your body with more calories than what's required to maintain the reduced physical state, then your body will begin storing excess energy, which leads to an accumulation of fat tissue. It's a constant balancing act.

To maintain your muscle mass, include 150 to 300 minutes of moderate intensity physical activity and two or more days of strength training per week.[2] Cardio exercises you can do at home to keep your muscles active and your body limber include: high knees, mountain climbers, cross jacks, burpees, stair sprints, squats, push-ups, planks, lunges.

GYM TALK

As a seasoned trainer with over four decades' experience, I have tested hundreds of high intensity training methods and my favoured technique for building lean muscle is dropsets.

The dropset technique is to repeat an exercise at a certain weight or level until you reach fatigue and then reduce that weight or level and continue with more repetitions (and more 'drops') until you reach muscle failure at each level. This is also known as the multi-poundage system, discovered in 1947 by Henry Atkins.

WHY DO BODYBUILDERS LOVE DROPSETS?

When you work in sets you are only recruiting a certain number of muscle fibres at each set. As you drop the weight down and continue, you engage different muscle fibres, which promotes better muscle growth than sticking with the same weight.

Studies have shown regular dropset training for over 50s can improve muscle mass, muscle strength, muscle endurance and most important of all, greater functionality, which becomes a priority as you move into your 60s, 70s and beyond.[3] Dropset usage can increase the muscle hypertrophic response to resistance training.[4] Regular training will increase your chances at longevity!

DON'T FORGET TEMPO

The concept of tempo is another important element you can add to your repertoire to keep your training engaging and fun. Tempo is the name for the timing and delivery of the components of your specific exercise and is usually seen as a 3 or 4 number code. Some people like to explode their weights upwards; others like slow, steady long holds, each method will have a different tempo. For example, someone learning to lift might begin with a 4-1-2-1 tempo as outlined below.

4 – negative movement or lowering the weight
1 – pause
2 – muscle tension rising to meet the resistance of the exercise or lift
1 – pause

As you improve and adapt your training, the first pause may become a zero so as to explode up into the lift. Exercising with rep tempos allows you to carefully manage (and maximise) your time under tension — which is our objective — to contract and work the muscles to achieve hypertrophy: the increase or refining of our targeted muscles.

Exercising with tempo has great benefits such as improved stability and body control and it's a good way to develop connective tissue, which is important for those starting out.

Take a look at my tempo video at leanmuscle.com.

IIIII

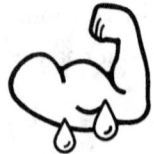

LET'S SWEAT

Now that you have read some of the important foundations about body and nutrition and you can recognise the excuses, it's time to get your blood pumping and start sweating! I have listed some exercises here that you can try.

These following ten exercises will induce sweating by using your own body weight. You will not need any extra equipment, nor require much space and you can be barefoot so there really is no excuse not to start *now*. They can be done anywhere and anytime.

If you are in doubt, speak with your health professional to make sure you are able to partake in the physicality of the exercises, and make sure you do not overexert yourself and cause injury. Don't start with all guns blazing; take it slowly.

When you begin, start with what is comfortable for you. Your goal is to get your heart rate up and start sweating. I recommend holding each for 15–30 second intervals. This will vary according to your personal fitness.

Pike Push-ups	The pike push-up is different to the standard push up. It targets the shoulders and chest, and helps to counter body weakness and develop muscle over the whole body.
	• Take a normal push-up position on the floor. Make sure your arms are straight and your hands are shoulder width apart. Now, lift your hips to form an upside down V. Keep your arms and legs as straight as possible.
	• Bend your elbows until your head is almost touching the floor, pause for a moment and then lift yourself back up.
Handstand Push-ups	This is a great test of your upper body strength.
	• Get yourself in a handstand position – use the wall if necessary.
	• Lower yourself to the floor, keeping your elbows in front of your shoulders. Get as low as you can and then push up again.
Bear Crawl	One of my favourites – this uses the strength in the shoulders and is a bodyweight mobility exercise. It also uses the strength in the quads and abdominals. The bear crawl is similar to the baby crawl but you are on your hands and toes to hold the weight of your body.

Frog Squats (actually *these* are my favourite)	• Stand upright with your feet a little wider than shoulder-width apart. • Hold your hands out in front of your body at arm's length. • Squat until your thighs are parallel to the floor and you can touch the floor. • Inhale while squatting. • Exhale while pushing yourself back up into the standing position.
Plank	• Start on the ground. Place your hands directly under your shoulders. • Step your feet back (similar to push up stance). To gain more stability, keep your feet hip-distance apart. To challenge yourself, keep your feet closer together. • Keep your body in a straight line from your feet to your head. Hold this position while you tighten your abdominal muscles, your glutes and quads.
Renegade Row	• In a push up position, balance all of your weight on your feet. Keep your feet about shoulder length apart. • Pull one arm up toward your torso keeping it close, until the elbow is just behind the torso. • Lower the hand to the ground and pull the other hand back. Then repeat. • To challenge yourself, use weights as you pull your hands up. • Check out the relevant video at leanmuscle.com.

EXERCISES

Glute Bridge	• Lay down on your back. Bend your knees and keep your feet flat on the floor. • Lift your hips off the ground until your knees and shoulders align into a straight line. • Squeeze those glutes in tightly and keep your abs drawn in and tight. This will ensure you don't overextend your back.
Prone Back Extension	• On your stomach on the floor, extend your legs fully. • Bring your arms into a back extension. • Engage and tighten your back muscles. • Pause and hold and return to a relaxed position. Repeat.
Bodyweight Squat	This is a great squat to maintain lower-body strength. • Stand with your feet about shoulder width apart. • Keep your back in a natural state. Your weight should be spread to your feet as you squeeze into the squat. • When you lift yourself back up, keep your knees in line with your feet, and make sure your feet are facing forward (not inward).
The Overhead Lunge	This is a great way to strengthen your lower body and build balance. • This is literally a normal lunge, with your arms raised above your head.

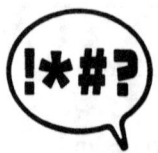

PERMISSION TO SWEAR

Here, I have listed the top ten exercises (these exercises include weights) that are sure to make you swear. Enjoy!

Dips
- Support yourself on the bars with your elbows locked and your hands turned out (for added support use a resistance band and rest on your knees — this will help you maintain safety and ensure good form).
- Keep a long neck and shoulders slightly forward to begin.
- Slowly extend down until your shoulder is just below the elbow.
- Press up and finish back in elbow lock position
- To minimise the pressure on your shoulders, contract your upper back by pinching your shoulder blades together.

Deadlift

Deadlifts are a great exercise because they are very challenging. This is a great one if you have knee issues.

- Stand with your feet hip width apart.
- Holding the barbell in front of your shins, keep your hips and lower chest hinged and facing the ground. Push up through your heels, thrusting your hips forward (for beginners use a hex-bar whereby you hold the barbell with palms facing inwards).
- Maintain a flat back and keep your core tight. Pause, lower and repeat.

Check out the relevant video at leanmuscle.com.

Dumbbell Thruster	An awesome core stabilizing exercise, which challenges your whole body, improving flexibility in your hips and shoulders whilst building strength.

- Form your arms in a bicep curl holding a pair of dumbbells (whatever weight you can manage).
- Keep your elbows bent and bring the weights right up to your face.
- Push arms straight up ahead, standing tall, arms fully extended over your shoulder. Squeeze your quads, abs and glutes while doing this.
- Come back down into a full squat while lowering the dumbbells back again so that the bottom of the squat and the dumbbells are back into the starting position.

The Bench Press	- Lie flat on your back on a bench with your eyes directly under the bar. Lift your chest and squeeze through your shoulder blades. Your feet should remain flat on the floor.
- Grab hold of the bar and place your little finger on the knurl or ring of the bar. Wrap your palms around the bar. Keep wrists down and obtain a full grip.
- Inhale and on the exhale, press (lift) the bar and straighten your arms, lifting the bar slightly over your shoulders with your elbows locked.
- Keeping your elbows tucked in and your forearms vertical, lower the bar to your mid chest and hold your breath a moment at the bottom of the movement.
- Repeat from the exhale, remembering to keep your buttocks firmly on the bench.

The Barbell Row	• Keep your lower back neutral to prevent any injury or pain. Do not round your spine. • Rest the bar on the floor between reps to prevent injury. • Rows place a lot of pressure on the back and arms so start with low weights and gradually increase according to your strength.
One Arm Kettlebell Press	Dumbbells can be used if you do not have kettlebells. • Stand with feet shoulder width apart and the kettlebell placed in front of your right foot. • On ascent and descent, be sure to maintain a stable, neutral spine position. Put your left hand on the small of your back and only use your right hand/arm to start with. • Keep your buttocks down and your palm facing your body. • With your right arm fully extended, keep your core tight, lifting the kettlebell bringing it up to your shoulder, all the while keeping your chest tight and using your heels to lift. • Continue to lift the weight up with your arm extended over your head. Keep the kettlebell close to your body. When you bring it overhead, rotate your wrist so that your palm is facing forward. • Restrict any back movement or arching and keep back straight. • Lower the kettlebell back to your shoulder with control and repeat. Check out the relevant video at leanmuscle.com.

EXERCISES

Pull-Up — To enhance your upper body strength, the pull up is a great exercise to incorporate into your exercise routine. You can have a wide grip, a tight grip or close grip. Each one of these will consider different challenges.

- Keep your core tight. Squeeze your glutes as you pull up and grip the bar as tightly as you can (for beginners: secure a resistance band on top of the chin bar and place the balls of your feet on the band, this will ensure proper form and control).
- To up the challenge, grip a small weight plate with your feet as you pull yourself up.

The Turkish Get Up

- Lay on your back on the floor with a kettlebell next to your right side. Roll slightly towards it.
- Grab the kettlebell with two bent arms (make sure you use both arms) and roll back onto your back, firmly holding the kettlebell.
- Let go of the kettlebell with your left hand.
- Bench press with your right arm, keeping your arm vertical and locked.
- Bend your right knee and firmly place your foot on the ground.
- Lift your right shoulder off the floor – support your weight with left elbow and hand until your left arm is straight.
- Raise your buttocks and extend your left leg off the floor.
- Pass your left leg underneath and pause with your left knee on the ground beneath your torso. The kettlebell is still raised above your head in the locked position.
- Stand up and hold that position then return to the starting position again by doing all the steps in reverse.
- Set a timer starting with 5 minutes, working your way up to 15 minutes, then change sides.

| Bicep Curl | • Stand with your back straight holding a dumbbell in each hand. Keep your arms hanging by your sides.
• Keep your elbows close to your torso and your palms should be facing forward. Your upper arms should be stationary the whole time.
• Exhale as you curl up, then inhale as you bring your dumbbell down. The weights should be curled up to shoulder level when contracting biceps. |
|---|---|

You might notice how often I incorporate the kettlebell into my exercises. I have a fascination and respect for this piece of equipment and couldn't train without it in fact. The kettlebell has been around for 300 years and was first used in Russia as a counterweight to weigh their crops. Kettlebell training builds powerful forearms, a strong grip and strong mind and muscle connections. Kettlebells possess a thicker handle than their barbell and dumbbell counterparts, so they really tax your grip, which develops greater forearm strength. As our society continues to move away from manual labour, grip strength continues to decrease as well, so we need to give it special attention in our workouts. They provide a well-rounded workout as long as you have sufficient understanding of their weight distribution and propensity for swing motions. I love sharing the benefits of this simple piece of workout equipment that enables great results.

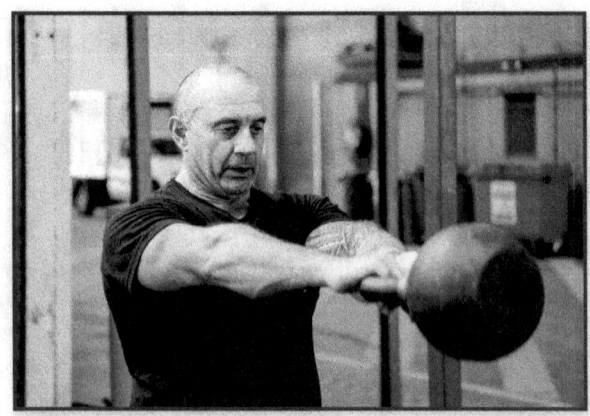

HOW TO GET THAT SIX-PACK

The most common questions I get asked are about how to attain a set of six-pack abdominals. As with everything, it requires dedication and hard work. Many people crunch away to no results and eventually find they've made common mistakes such as training their abs every day, sometimes 3 or 4 times a day.

Here are some hints for achieving that six-pack:
- More cardio to burn belly fat – activities such as running, walking, biking, swimming or more of your favourite sport are easy ways to fit cardio into your day.
- Increase muscle mass through exercises that engage abdominal muscles such as squats, deadlifts, swings, crunches, bridges and planks.
- Increase your protein intake and ensure your nutrition plan safeguards your metabolism and muscle mass during your weight loss phrase.
- Increase your heart rate and burn calories through High Intensity Interval Training (HIIT).

Richard is a great example of what you can achieve with discipline and hard work. Check out his story in Chapter 7.

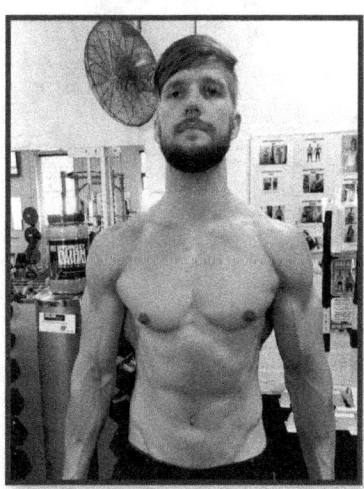 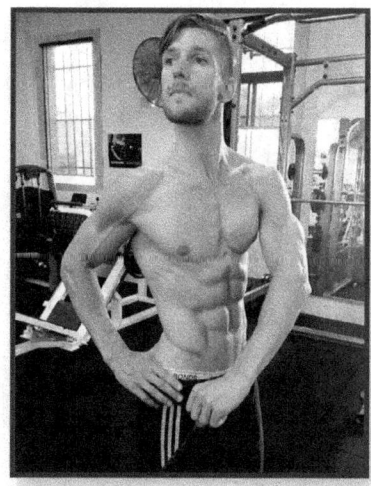

Remember the key is consistency, stay the course and your shape will begin changing. One last thing...don't forget to *Smile*!

PERMISSION TO SMILE

So often I see people going through their fitness journey without enough fun in their training. They forget to have fun along the way, especially when their old beliefs come back to haunt them. Often they relive the last time they tried to lose weight and they remember struggling not smiling.

Yes, it will require you to roll up your sleeves, but that doesn't mean you can't do it without fun along the way. You're exposing yourself to a whole new set of learnings when you join me that carry forward with you in all aspects of your life. It's like you're finally starting your new life that you were always meant to live. How cool is that!

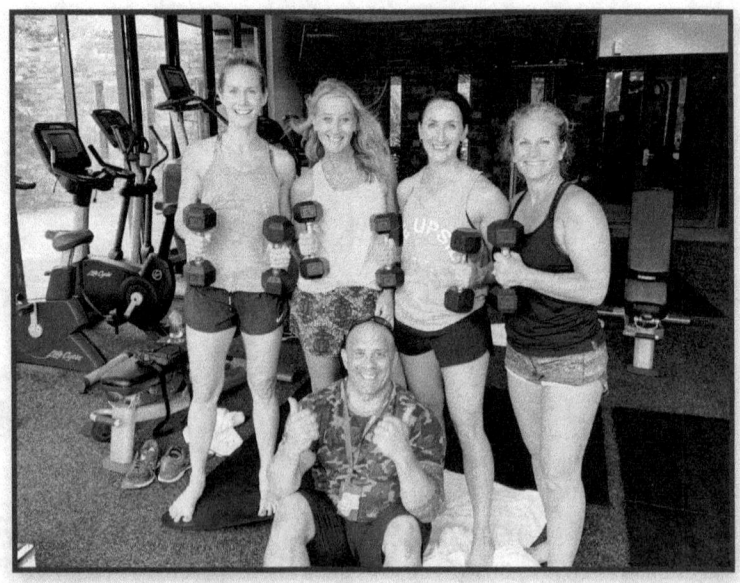

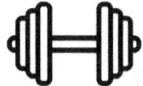

CHAPTER 6

WORKOUT

SKYROCKET YOUR JOURNEY

Many times I have seen people who are struggling or have struggled all their life to get lasting results. And I recognise there is a trend when it comes to fitness and most people feel inadequate in their ability to get the results they want when they're at the start of the road. They think; *I could never do that.* But I'm here to tell you; you can, if you start at the right place.

Rather than being a short-term solution, fitness is a lifelong resolution and commitment that produces lifelong benefits but it must start somewhere. It has to move out of your thought zone into action zone. It starts with you digging deep for the courage to find and choose a personal trainer to teach you how to move, how to target and match your nutrition to your goals, how and when to train, how to keep your mind sharp, focused and motivated and how to stretch, revisit and improve your goals.

Remember the 'what-why-how' we spoke about earlier in Chapter 2? There is nothing that makes me prouder than when I witness the steely focus of my clients' progress, they become intent on reaching their goals and their inner strength takes over; and my job is done. It is incredibly rewarding for both of us!

GET A GRIP

I remember as a kid my uncle used to shake my hand in greeting. He was a brickie with a super strong grip, grabbing onto those heavy bricks all day like they were nothing. I would watch him shake hands with my father too and I began to understand the importance of a grip firstly from a cultural perspective. It was a simple gesture but spoke volumes about strength and friendship and humility. I would practise shaking both their hands until my hands were so sore I couldn't do anymore handshaking.

From there I learnt a long time ago your grip strength was key to getting certain movements done, like pulling movements such as chin-ups in the park or hanging off a swing. As a kid we would see how long we could hang from a tree branch until our forearms gave way (I always won that game!).

Similar to the growing pattern where people often neglect their legs while working out, many people also neglect other smaller body parts in the misconception that these body parts add no value to their goals.

When was the last time you really shook someone's hand and checked their grip strength? When did you last train your forearms? It could be what is holding you back from becoming a full-blown beast in the weight room (if that's your goal). This is evident in the modern fad around ninja warrior competition courses you see on TV. The big muscly competitors' grips often fail them at crucial times while the people with rock-climbing experience excel with their grip strength and stamina to hold their own body weight!

Indirectly, grip strength develops in a number of common exercise movements:

- Crushing Grip – closing your hand and squeezing something, such as a dumbbell.

- Pinching Grip – holding an object between your thumb and another finger, and just squeezing with your fingertips.
- Supporting Grip – supporting an object with a crush grip, while your fingers take most of the load, like carrying a heavy bucket.
- Open Crush Grip – a crush grip where your fingers do not overlap, they are spread apart as in opening a jar.

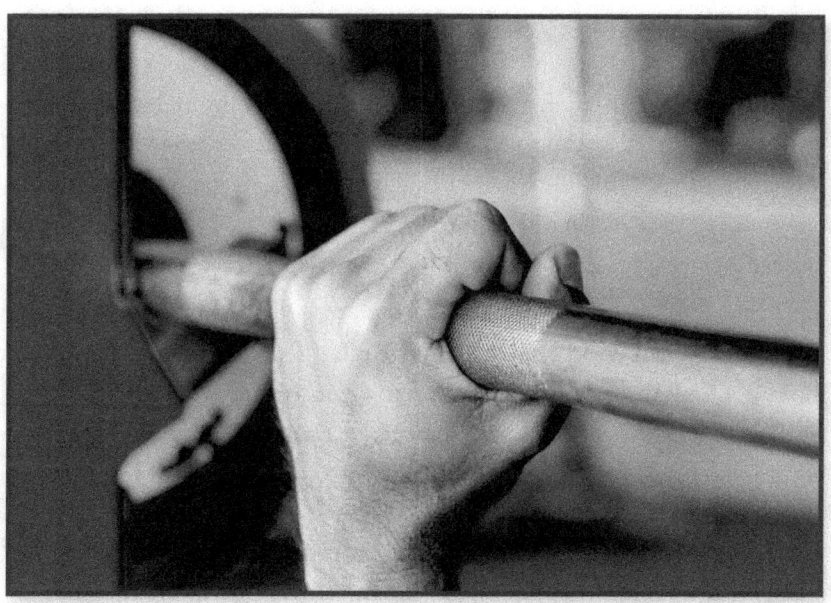

The good news is that your grip strength keeps improving the more you train however, if the goal here is to accelerate your grip strength then you need to focus on a few direct movements. Here are my 3 favourites:

For beginners – Farmer's Walk:
Carry a kettlebell in each hand (or even dumbbells) and slowly walk with your core tight (brace for impact), your neck muscles low (not raising your shoulders), keep your body compact (brace for impact) and feel the burn.

For intermediates – Barbell Dead Hangs:
Set a loaded bar up in a squat rack, with the height of the bar being just a few inches under where you would lock out in a deadlift. Grab the bar with a double overhand grip at shoulder width, keep the bar away from touching you too much and stand tall, hold for 15-30 seconds. Repeat for sets and reps.

For more advanced – Dead Hangs on a chin-up bar:
Choose a secure bar and position a box under your feet so you don't go injuring yourself. Even better is to ask someone to stand close by and they can also time you. Hold onto the bar and hang your body weight off it. This also helps stretch out and decompress the spine. Work your way up in duration to prevent injury and be sure not to sway; dead hang means dead still.

I once trained a bodybuilder who couldn't do one chin-up without the aid of gloves and straps. He actually used them for nearly every workout during his gym sessions and his forearms had not developed and his grip strength was sub-par for his size. I promised him I would improve his size and strength in nearly every body part.

His grip would fail before his muscles did on exercises like pull-ups and the dead-lift. Just like training for other body parts, he'd deprived his forearms of the basic training needed for growth. This guy couldn't even hold a pair of dumbbells without his hands hurting. I explained he was only as strong as his grip and changes needed to be made.

Firstly, to develop his grip he really had to remove the gloves or straps on all of his lifts. We began focussing on his forearm training to make it seem like he had bigger wrists. Using this mindset, he sucked it up and started lifting without gloves or straps. The first week or so his hands were callused and bleeding like hell. I was fair but firm when I told him to, "Quit complaining, it will be worth it in the end, I promise you."

He needed to let his hands adapt to the new feeling of fresh skin grinding against the iron. Under no circumstances did I let his hands touch gloves or straps. To his credit, he kept up a strong attitude and it became habitual. One month later his forearms looked nearly twice the size and his grip strength had improved dramatically.

I am not suggesting that straps should never be used under any circumstances. Regardless of whether your muscles can handle more weight than your grip, your body acts as a unit. So your muscle strength and growth will be curtailed by wearing gloves between the skin and the bar.

If your grip continues to be at a severe disadvantage and you are much stronger than your hands are even after working on your grip, then it would be acceptable to use straps only for heavy compound movements and one intense set, such as dead-lifts, pull-ups, or bent-over rows.

Nevertheless, your best bet is to do what I did from day one and stick to chalk rather than straps, since it more closely replicates a natural grip. Train your forearms as if it were any other body part. You wouldn't neglect your chest, would you? A good way to get a forearm workout in is to do one or two sets at the end of your workout. Note also with forearms, you want to do extremely high reps.

One of the best exercises (and my favourite) I give clients for forearms is the one I explained earlier, the Farmer's Walk with kettlebells. Set aside one set at the end of your workout in which you take the walk to complete failure (the feeling in your forearms where the lactic acid builds up so severely that you feel like you can't go on for another second). Work your forearms out a maximum of three times a week, but not on consecutive days.

BAREFOOT WORKOUT

It's worth a reminder from the previous chapter that it's time to ditch the shoes because it does not serve your higher purpose. I find it to be a fantastic feedback mechanism – training barefoot allows me to see what my clients are doing with their feet and ankles while they are lifting and ensuring they have good form. If you are training alone, check your form in the mirror or just record your movement on your phone, be it a short video for example.

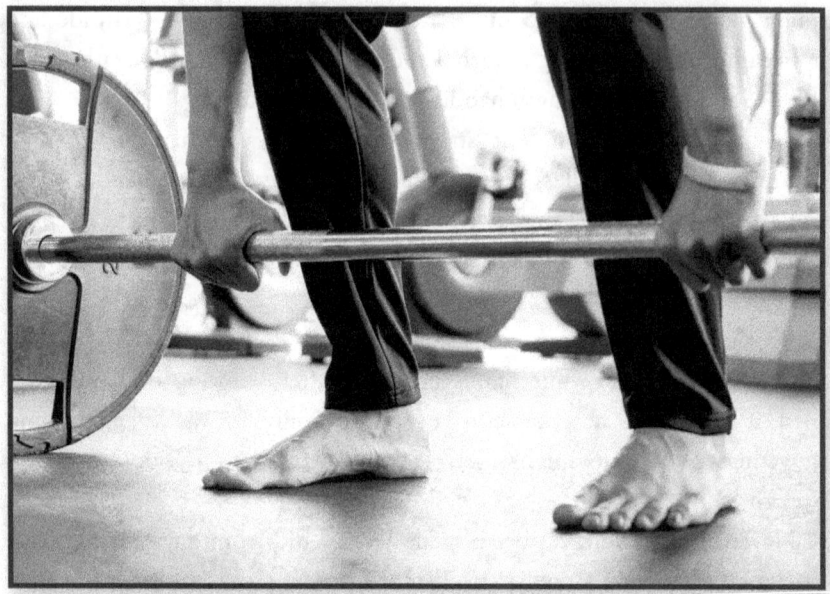

Nothing feels better than training barefoot; that sense of freedom it gives you and the connection with the ground. We don't often use the ground to our advantage. By exercising barefoot, you can actually promote your sense of balance, improve muscle alignment, reduce orthopaedic pains, and lessen the chance of injury. Just as our biceps need flexing to build muscle, so do our toes.

KEEP IT REAL

I can tell you that I am a constant work in progress and have been on the quest of developing a lean body and strong muscles since the early '80s. From firsthand experience I know that to gain strength and size, you have to push and overload your muscles beyond their capacity. Yes, you need to feel the burn but without sacrificing the form, always go for progression and if you do it without sacrificing form you will have a much better chance!

CARDIO TYPES

There are two types of cardio: low impact and high impact. If weight loss is your goal, I strongly suggest a combination of both. From experience I would often perform a high impact session such as sprinting once a week. The quick burst of energy and elevated feeling you get makes sprinting a great choice. I have always enjoyed sprinting. Even as a teenager I was always on the lookout for the highest hill to run up then walk down (this contributed to my leg development).

You get into low impact cardio before and after strength training. Working out on a treadmill with a slight incline and speed set to 5, wearing a weighted vest for 45-60 minutes will certainly get the results you want. Another benefit of low impact cardio is it gives you the chance to think about your personal goals and the workout you are invested in.

RAISE YOUR LIMITS SENSIBLY

A problem I have seen many times over the years is when someone trains to muscle failure; it often leads to overtraining, injuries and increased recovery times. Repetitious training to muscle failure only trains your body to failure, then lifting to your max only meets your limits; it doesn't raise them.

What you should do is train to expand your comfort zone. This way your body adapts to change in a sensible manner so don't focus on lifting huge weights for extremely low reps, focus on optimising your training with small increments of weight over a longer period of time.

If you think there is a magic pill or potion you are misled, don't get reeled into that hype.

PREVENTING INJURIES

New injuries can be avoided and existing injuries can be managed with the right tools and approaches to individual exercises. As a personal trainer, I am able to explain how to prevent injuries, teach the correct techniques and ensure you have a good understanding before trying it out, together we can really minimise the risk of injury to almost zero.

Educate yourself about the differing muscles and how to work them safely and effectively for maximum impact. Always remain hydrated. I know I say it a lot in every situation but your body needs water, period. If you fail to remain properly hydrated, you can end up lightheaded, your muscles can fatigue prematurely, and you can impact your body's ability to cool down through perspiration.

Maintain regular visits with a physiotherapist or chiropractor to 'tune' your body back into alignment. These health professionals will also be able to perform muscle and joint testing and identify any areas of the body that are underperforming and need more attention.

When working out make sure you are wearing light and loose clothing so that you are free to move in various directions and positions without causing too much strain.

Stretching and cooling down is important in reducing injuries – this is an area individuals often skip, thinking they don't really need to do it. Remember that Rome wasn't built in a day…and neither will that incredible body of yours! Be patient and learn the right techniques so that you can continue to work out and enjoy a healthy and fit body.

Our bodies are truly remarkable in terms of the feedback they give us. When we have injuries or any kind of inflammation, our bodies go into action defending an area to protect it. We need to listen to what it's telling us.

YOUR OWN BODY WEIGHT

Unlike the '80s, we now have a whole lot of gadgets and training aids at our fingertips. Some belong in the rubbish tip, others belong in the gym, but right off the bat I can tell you the best training apparatus is your own body weight.

As a growing boy I recall being fascinated by the gymnasts at the Olympic Games, how symmetrical their bodies looked. Every inch of their body had been trained equally, allowing them to send their body weight flying easily through the air. Gymnasts train using a lot of bodyweight exercises. Body weight training has been around for centuries and can be done anywhere and anytime so it has many advantages.

Even the most advanced athletes would find it hard to do a full body workout for 30 minutes.

Here are some easy ways to alter your exercises to use more of your bodyweight:
- Altering the leverage i.e. feet-elevated push-ups vs. standard push-ups
- Changing the weight-to-limb ratio i.e. pistol squats vs. lunges
- Increasing the range of motion i.e. pull-ups to chest vs. pull-ups to chin.

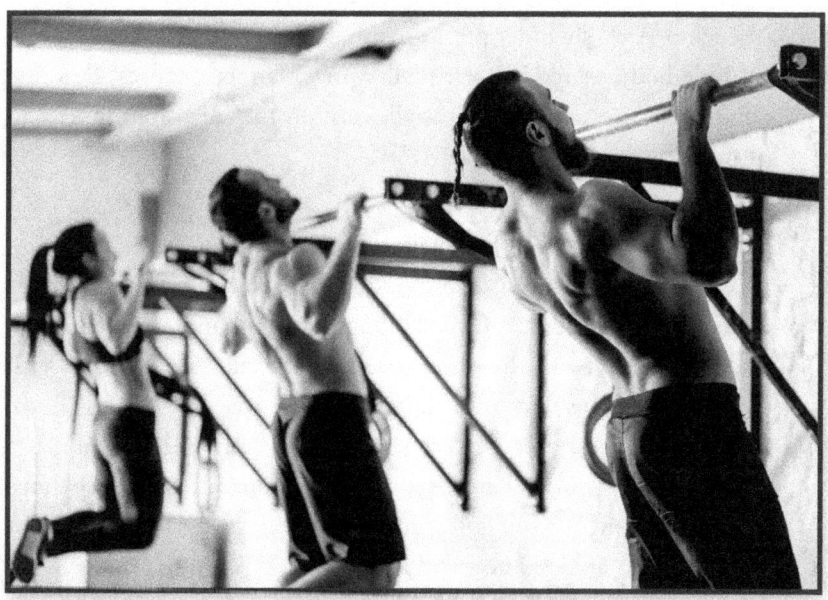

TRAIN YOUR ENTIRE BODY

It can be said you are only as tough as your weakest leak so it stands to reason that when you push your body to the edge of failure, it is your weakest link that will most likely suffer the injury.

Training isolated muscles does have its place, just think of bodybuilders who are looking for aesthetic results, however for most people most of the time, it's important to train the muscles to work together; it's about shifting your mindset to utilise the whole kinetic chain of the body.

Through total body conditioning, you're more likely to be injury free. Don't skip leg day just cause it burns a bit, switch up your activities to engage all muscle groups in a kinetic chain to develop weak links.

Here are some ideas on strengthening through the kinetic chain:
- Hamstrings flexibility – downward dog to engage feet, calves, hamstrings, glutes and lower back all at once.
- Greater leg strength and muscle – squats and deadlifts (both double and single leg versions), kettlebell swings, lunges, and step-ups.
- Stronger arms – pull-ups, chin-ups, seated and bent over rows; and pushing with the whole chain vertically and horizontally – push-ups, bench presses, shoulder presses, push presses.
- Whole body exercise – kettlebell swings, farmer's carries, deadlifts, suitcase carries and ball slams all work on the core, and upper and lower body.

Here are some suggestions for total-body conditioning:
- Compound your exercises by working multiple muscles with a single exercise e.g. combine a forward lunge with holding a kettlebell and adding a core twist, then do a reverse lunge and side lunges as well. Hit all directions to achieve muscle balance over time.
- Stay single – do exercises using your own body weight while also maintaining your balance e.g. single-leg presses, single-leg hops, single-leg lunges. You'll see an increase in strength and stability around your ankles, knees and hips.
- Add one or two total-body plyometric exercises (squat jumps, lunges) and interval (sprint) workouts each week to maintain a balance between fast and slow-twitch fibres (how fast or slow the fibres are to contract).

On my website leanmuscle.com you'll find some technique videos. In the 12-Week Challenge, I have built an extensive library of exercises explaining the right technique for the right equipment and how to use it all the right way in order to gain excellent outcomes.

MIND BODY CONNECTION

There is a saying amongst old school bodybuilders like myself, "Put your mind in the muscle." I recall when I was in a locker room once, getting ready for a workout I noticed my chest could flex and contract with a thought. I thought what a great party trick so I started flexing and contracting my biceps.

In other words, I was putting my mind in the muscle; it was a conscious and deliberate muscle contraction that I stumbled upon. Then I had the ability to focus the tension during exercise on a specific muscle group, like flexing the chest in between sets as I still do nowadays; it's a great reminder of that connection we often overlook.

Are you connecting the dots between thoughts and actions? Make your brain the biggest muscle of all when working out. It is crucial that when you are training, you think, visualise and connect with the movement. If you are performing a shoulder press, you must consider the stability of your shoulders, keeping a strong frame and gripping the weights with just the right amount of pressure. The movement, as with Tai Chi, must become one with your mind and part of you as a whole. Having this strong connection with the movements and the routine will establish great muscle movement, growth and flexibility.

CHECK YOURSELF BEFORE YOU WRECK YOURSELF

These days people are juggling so many things trying to fit everything in and we're not present in the moment or present with our body. Before exercising I recommend (and I mean every time), taking a moment to check-in with your body and mind:

- How is your energy?
- What is your mood?
- How does your body feel? Are there any places you're storing stress, tension, or emotion?

Knowing this, ask yourself what kind of exercise is right for you today?
- Should you start with a few exercises to boost your energy?

- Or a hard cardio workout to burn off stress?
- Or a strength workout to feel grounded?
- Or some functional movements to address muscular imbalances?

By noticing how your body and mind feels in the moment, you can choose a workout that meets your needs. If you are feeling tired and are not quite sure if you should or should not workout, give it a few minutes. Start slow, ease into it, and check in with how you feel. Sometimes a workout can completely transform your energy and turn you from sleepy to energizer bunny.

Sometimes it does not work that way. It's always worth getting moving for 10 minutes to see how it goes. If you feel good and end up exercising for longer then that's great. If not, at least you achieved some movement and found out how your body feels. It is always worth it to try a few minutes and check in with your physical self.

Be mindful of motivational fitness quotes. Ones that target your mind and soul are inspiring. Stay away from the body shaming types such as, "Push through the pain," or, "Don't stop unless you puke, faint or pass out." Crazy I know, but I've heard it all. These mantras will end up hurting you physically and ultimately mentally as well.

When shopping around for a fitness class, if the instructor pressures or pushes you to compromise your health to 'conquer' a workout, it's not a supportive or healthy choice. Find a trainer who will help you challenge yourself in a positive way, growing your mental strength as well.

DO NOT SACRIFICE FORM OVER WEIGHT

If your technique or form is incorrect, not only is your progress going to be significantly delayed or halted but you are inviting injury. Too often I see individuals perform a deadlift with little or no understanding of the technique, which is a must to minimise the impact on the body.

I have witnessed cases where a person needed to go for ACL surgery, rotator cuff repair, or fix a herniated disc in their back, all because of their failure to learn and maintain proper technique. If you are not sure, hire a trainer; after all we are in it for the benefit of all. Weigh up the cost of hiring a trainer for a single session of technique practice versus a lifetime of pain and allied care due to an injury sustained through incorrect form.

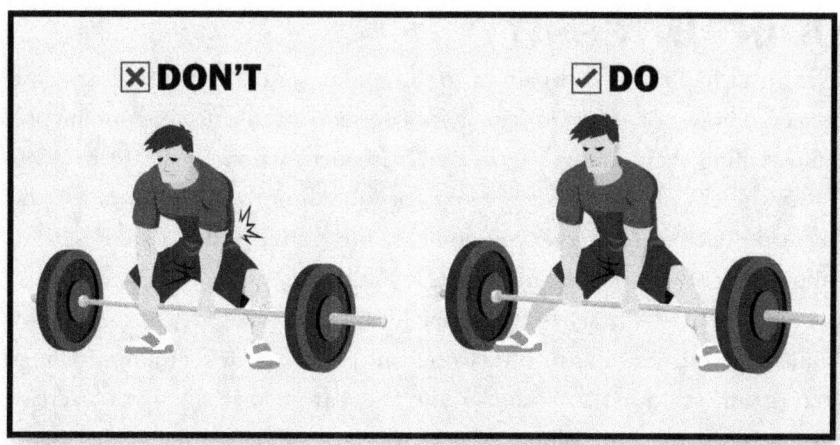

When you exercise, you must think and focus, instead of mindlessly repeating the motions or concentrating on just getting the weight up. You are there to work out the specific muscle you are targeting and that requires training it with deliberation and care. At the beginning and end of every repetition, pause and squeeze the muscles you are exercising, the mind and muscle must connect!

Never use the momentum of the swing to lift the weights nor let gravity drop the weight. Control the weight on the way down, spending as much time on the eccentric phase of the movement as on the concentric, therefore you must lift and lower the weight slowly, feeling the tension in your muscles while resisting the load the entire time.

For muscles to receive the impetus to grow, you have to stress them to the maximum by creating a proper stimulus. This only happens when you overload the muscle. But in order to do this, you need to go heavy enough and do enough repetitions, until you feel you cannot go any further without sacrificing good form. You'll come to recognise this degree within yourself.

If you go too heavy and use poor form, you incorporate other muscles that are not intended to be worked on by the exercise you are doing. As a result, you fail to sufficiently stimulate the targeted muscle to respond by repairing the muscle fibres to come back stronger. Progressive overload is what forces your muscles to grow, and can be achieved by increasing the weight or number of reps completed each successive week.

JOINT INTEGRITY

We've all had aches and pains at one time or another whether it's in the knees, elbows, or other joints. It's a common problem faced by anyone undertaking their strength goals and a frequent comment heard in gyms everywhere. "My knees are so sore" or "I've been on painkillers for the ache in my elbow", and yet you don't see this problem discussed or written about very often in fitness magazines.

Small short-term aches can generally be self-managed and assisted by adjusting your training to suit. I do want to point out that chronic long-term pain is another story and if you suffer from that when you exercise you should seek professional advice from a good sports medicine doctor to ascertain the deeper problem. Resist the self-diagnosis that could potentially injure yourself further or it could stop you from living a full and active life.

For joint integrity remember to:
- Warm up adequately
- Don't overtrain; too long or too often
- Don't overload; too much weight on low reps more often than you should
- Always take sufficient time off between workouts to allow muscles, tendons and joints to recover
- Use the correct form during heavy lifts
- Ensure your body is receiving adequate nutrients

WARM-UP AND FLEXIBILITY

Warming up gives your body time to adjust to the demands of exercise by putting you in a focused state, gets your blood flowing, raises your muscle temperature and increases your breathing rate.

The simplest way to warm up is an aerobic activity at an easy pace. How long you spend warming up will depend on your fitness level. If you are newer to exercise, your body will respond better with a longer warm up.

When warming up choose stretches that can be done standing up. Floor stretches are best for your cool down segment.

WORKOUT LENGTH

Initially, if you are just starting out to improve your overall health, commence with 30–60 minutes of continuous, steady-state exercise up to three times a week. Then to increase the results and benefits, after a few weeks, train for a minimum of 45 minutes three times per week of higher intensity interval training.

It is important to listen to your body for feedback – if your muscles are sore, dial it back to a light to medium workout then scale up the intensity when you feel ready. Do some light, fun activities in between the heavy workout days to keep your fitness levels up. Stretching while watching TV or a long walk with the dog are great additions to any routine.

RESTS BETWEEN SETS

Rest periods really range according to the exercise being performed. If you are doing squats or deadlifts (a compound movement) rest periods should not last more than 3 minutes. For isolation exercises like bicep curls and lateral raises, a good rest is 30 seconds to a minute at the most. You want to keep it at high intensity through the workout to gain the most out of it. We go into more depth about intensity and rests between sets in the 12-Week Challenge.

DON'T PUSH THROUGH THE PAIN

Remember, if it hurts — *stop!* Your body is a very powerful feedback system so listen to it. If you feel tired, do less. I let my energy levels and body awareness dictate how hard I work. While I love hard workouts (that make me sweat, swear and smile), I do not tackle maximal, high-intensity workouts *every* single session, no way.

When my body feels low on energy, I take that as a sign I need to go easier that day so I slow down and do exercises that make me feel good, and reassess whether to continue or focus on recovery with foam rolling for example. Using this strategy allows you to take care of yourself, stay active and make fitness a habit but without overdoing it.

COOLING DOWN

Cooling down after a workout helps with blood flow and allows for the gradual recovery of the pre exercise heart rate and blood pressure. It's important that you don't stop exercising abruptly. If your muscles suddenly stop contracting, this causes blood to accumulate in the lower extremities, and you'll lose blood pressure to pump it back to your heart and brain and you'll feel pretty dodgy. Always give yourself the opportunity to cool down.

FOAM ROLLERS

Why do they hurt so good? Foam rollers apply pressure to muscle fibres and the tissue surrounding the muscles, known as fascia (fibrous connective tissue). Muscle injury, inflammation or trauma can cause the tissue to bind to each other, lose elasticity, and form taut bands of tissue that can be painful.

Applying pressure and moving the fascia (myofascial release) can help separate these fibres and re-establish the integrity of the tissue. It is the nerve receptors activating within the muscles that gives you that feeling of release. If foam rolling is painful, you could be pressing too hard or have an existing injury that should be checked out by your health practitioner. Tennis balls and rolled up towels are other easy options to use for that muscle release and stretching.

At the end of the day, remember that just like any other workout recovery method, foam rolling should be used as a tool to help you feel better during and after workouts. That means that you can and should tweak your rolling habits until you find what works best for you. Forget about sticking to a strict schedule — start with rolling when you feel like you need it, or simply when you have time, and take it from there, depending on what feels right.

INJURY RECOVERY

We all get injuries from time to time; be it from a lapse in concentration when training or just an old existing injury coming to the surface. There are a few things that you can do and maintain to minimise your risk. Firstly, it pays to begin any fitness regime by getting the okay from your doctor after a full health check. This way you can do a follow-up health check in a few months' time to check how your health has improved; people's cholesterol often sees a big difference.

Once you get the all clear it is also important to keep your body in tune on a regular basis, I like to work with an osteopath. Osteopathy is a way of detecting, treating, and preventing health problems by moving, stretching, and massaging a person's muscles and joints. Osteopathy is based on the principle that the wellbeing of an individual depends on their bones, muscles, ligaments, and connective tissue functioning smoothly together.

Chiropractors treat and prevent mechanical disorders of the musculoskeletal system and the effects of these disorders on the function of the nervous system and general health. Chiropractors treat a range of musculoskeletal conditions, such as back pain, neck pain and headache.

Physiotherapy is treatment to restore, maintain, and make the most of a patient's mobility, function, and well-being. Physiotherapy helps through physical rehabilitation, injury prevention, and health and fitness. Physiotherapists get you involved in your own recovery.

So, remember when it comes to injury the goal should be to treat it straight away so it doesn't raise its ugly head. Don't forget to get a deep tissue massage when you feel the need too, they find the knots you didn't know you had!

Don't tough it out and force through the pain. Stop, evaluate your symptoms, and if needed take time off for healing and recovery. Don't be disheartened or reactive, leave your ego behind and use the time productively e.g. focus on your nutrition and meditation and make plans for your gradual recovery.

If injured, use RICE (Rest Ice Compression Elevation) to reduce swelling, alleviate pain and protect the injured area to accelerate the healing process. Never use heat on an acute injury (this increases blood flow and swelling), instead use ice to reduce the blood flow and swelling to injured tissue until you can seek medical attention.

LIGHTER WEIGHTS AND HIGHER REPS

I love training high volume at the best of times, however if you are training through an injury and working the affected area, use lighter weights and higher repetitions, though slower and more controlled. If done correctly, you can do gentle, frequent, low-intensity exercises with higher reps that can activate the muscles in the area and help the healing process. Especially if you have the injury diagnosed early and therefore, can start on your recovery straight away.

CHAPTER 7

CASE STUDIES

This book is all about results so it wouldn't be complete without presenting some more of the case studies I have worked with over the last few years. These individuals were happy to share our journeys together that show how focusing on fitness helps you not only achieve amazing results but also how it flows over into living a healthier, happier life.

Most of the case studies include a 'before' and 'after' shot. As I've mentioned, keeping visual records is one way of representing a person's physical changes and achievements. Many people find photos a great way to keep them accountable to their commitment while some people prefer to acknowledge their results privately. I thank the inspiring people for the stories that follow and I hope they resonate with you as they share their particular frustrations and challenges they faced in reaching their goal.

The goals were wide and varied; from wanting to loose weight, muscle up, be pain free, feel young again, gain confidence or to release those positive chemicals more often that make us feel good for longer. A couple of stories relate to the unseen benefits of health and fitness and their internal changes are just as inspiring.

In my experience, people come to me when they're finally ready to challenge themselves physically to see what they're capable of, it's usually something they have been dreaming about doing, something to tick off the bucket list in a way. They finally feel a driving force to really put the effort in, to give themselves a real opportunity for making changes that leaves no chance for regrets later in life. If this applies to you, I hope you're inspired to finally go after that dream too.

STACH

At 43 years old, Stach's weight had crept up to 155kg, which left him with very little energy and he found it hard to get out of bed in the morning. Stach wanted to see what he could achieve over 6-12 months of online training through my Lean Muscle program. Firstly, we started with recognising his daily habits before navigating a blueprint for a new nutrition plan to form new habits and setting small manageable goals to start with.

We also discussed his current beliefs (his story) about himself, his body and his mind. I gently challenged some of those beliefs that were holding him back. Together we wrote down an agenda going forward and a agreement that he felt comfortable with (but not too comfortable). Stach had to send me progress pictures, as he remained accountable for his own health and success whilst following my personal structure and formula for success. The pictures say it all!

Stach's goal was to shed 20 kilos, he achieved that and more, losing 41 kg over 12 months! It was a matter of going back to the drawing board, listening to his objections and working out what his true intent was for losing the weight.

As with many, Stach was a creature of habit, indulging in bad food and drink. I worked out an individualised plan for Stach as I do for all my clients and this is why they are all successful because they are all created around each client's needs.

In the words of Stach himself, *"Not only did I lose 41kgs of stubborn fat in less than 12 months with Master Coach Fred on his Lean Muscle Program, the program allowed me to accomplish what I thought was impossible.*

Fred even took the time to pick out healthy menu items on restaurant websites. I knew that this was no ordinary program and that he was 100% dedicated to my success. I soon saw something that I did not think existed – my waistline! Talk about feeling good about yourself. Life is different for me physically and mentally, and I owe it all to Fred!"

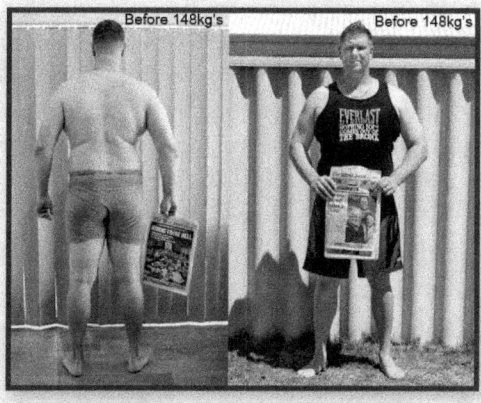

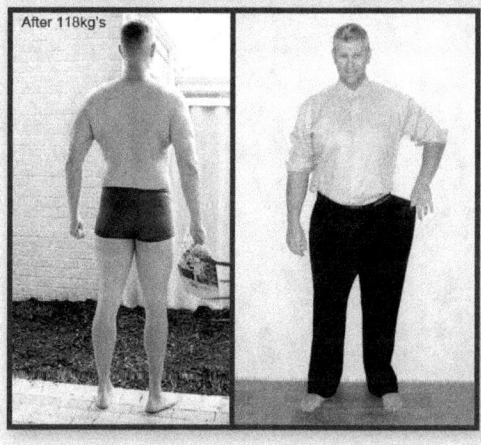

JOHN

John felt so out of shape, was overweight, slept poorly and he was in pain a lot. He wished he could feel fit again like in his younger days climbing monkey bars with ease. He didn't know where to begin, he knew his whole lifestyle would need a revamp and he was also concerned about injury and didn't know *how* to train.

John was a shift worker so had to commit to training at least 3 times a week no matter what. Once his clothes felt looser though he felt a real buzz for the first time and it was a good driving force to keep at it. John developed great muscle definition and was sleeping better than ever. John even achieved his goal of climbing on the monkey bars again; age is no barrier after all! From working with me, John said he learnt the importance of keeping within a healthy weight range and that you really need to *Sweat, Swear, Smile* every day! Check out John's Realfit transformation video at leanmuscle.com.

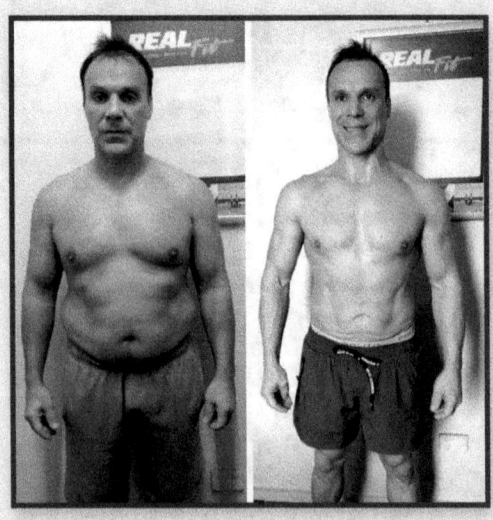

JAMES

James' career as an endocrine surgeon meant his schedule was very busy and his fitness had slipped over the years. He wanted to finally get that 6-pack and put muscle on his smaller frame. James made a big effort to make room for fitness in his busy life and was looking for the most results in an efficient time: that's where I came into the picture. I helped James create that blueprint that he needed to follow, especially with his nutrition and not cutting corners.

James improved quickly and had great potential to compete on stage, which he thought sounded exciting and challenging so he went for it! James was extremely happy to come 4th in the Fitness Model Novice category in the Victorian Natural Championships. It was an added accomplishment to his goal of not only getting fit but also achieving that elusive 6-pack. James said he learnt so much about training, nutrition and having a winner's mindset.

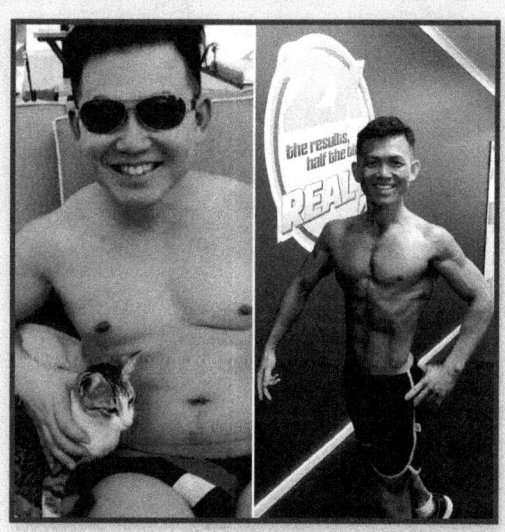

HANNAH

Hannah was in good shape when she contacted me. She was already training and boxing but she wanted to become leaner with the help of a good coach. Hannah admits she had a poor relationship with food and wasn't happy that she always seemed to feel tired. She wanted to be a fitness model on stage. I assured her it would happen so we had 19 weeks before her first show.

I created a blueprint for Hannah which enabled her to re-evaluate her relationship with food and she would cook up my easy recipes on a Sunday. Planning and prioritising were vital for Hannah. Progress pictures and regular measurements helped her stay accountable and along with a tough training program I asked her to send me photos of her food as well to check portion sizes. My 'traffic light system' really resonated with her too, especially when the going got tough.

Along with myself, Hannah said she had a lot of great support from family, friends and gym buddies that helped her believe in herself and her achievements and this spirit shone through in her fantastic stage presence on the big day. Hannah's advice is to, *"Find yourself a trainer that knows his sh*t! Fred brings out the best in my training and nutrition. Could not ask for a greater mentor."*

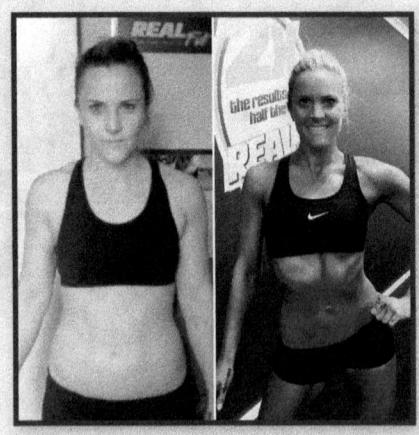

JESS

I had a unique experience in training my client Jess, who had a goal to one day win a fitness competition in the bikini division. I met her after she had returned from a fun gap year in Europe where she had first become fascinated with fitness competitions. While over there she enjoyed the good life and upon her return to Australia said she was in the worst shape of her life.

Jess found her own efforts at training and 'dieting' only gave her a narrow perspective to achieve the overall health, wellness and body she was looking for. She was disappointed at never progressing beyond a certain point. Jess also shared that she had always struggled with confidence and had battled an eating disorder for many years. She wanted to prove to herself that with the right coaching, she could achieve the body she wanted in a healthy way.

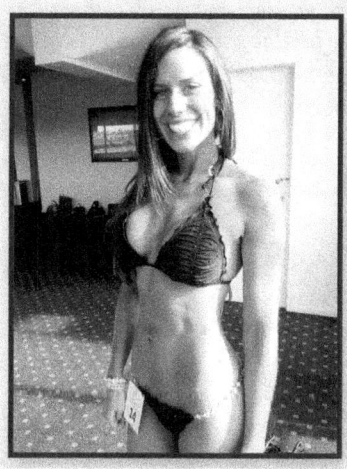 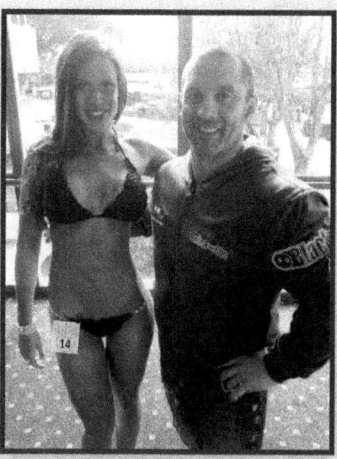

It was an amazing journey and this is what Jess said afterwards, *"Fred checked in with me 4 times a week and always encouraged me to move forward after I'd cheated on my nutrition. With his help over six months, I won my division in my very first competition. I moved from training to lose weight to training for the love of it. I learnt how important the right support is and also in my case, preparation, needing a set*

routine and regular meal prep. Many forms of therapy hadn't helped me overcome my challenges but Fred helped me learn to nurture my body in a healthy way."

MARGARITA

Margarita had a goal to get on stage in a bikini in her 40s. She was busy in work and family life and recognised she needed structured support and accountability. Margarita knew I would give her the best combination of training, nutrition and importantly mindset for whenever her doubts crept in. We worked together towards her goal over a 6-month period.

This is what Margarita had to say about her journey, *"I had known Fred from old school days' and he was into fitness back then. He always looked and walked the talk so to speak, so I knew Fred would give me that extra push I needed. His homework each week was a non-negotiable. I am always keeping fit and this transformation was a phenomenal part of my life. I was runner-up in the master's division and I learnt so much in the process."*

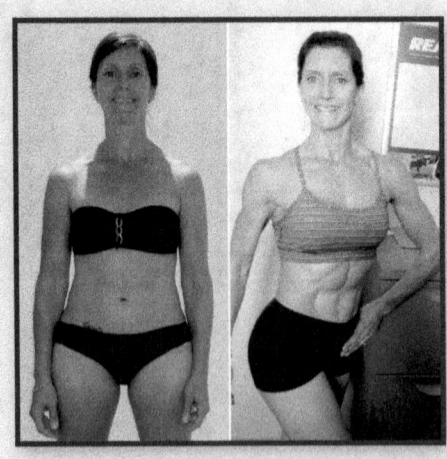

MILAN

Milan was frustrated that he was training hard but not seeing the results he was looking for. He was looking to learn new methods, wanted to look good and he had a goal of eventually becoming a Personal Trainer himself. His lack of knowledge was holding him back.

With no set timeframe in mind, Milan needed me to guide him and push his limits. He had the motivation but not the know-how. I showed him the importance of good nutrition and managing his calories which Milan admits was challenging but ultimately saw him succeed, proving to himself that with discipline, he could achieve his dream. Milan is now a successful PT himself in Sydney.

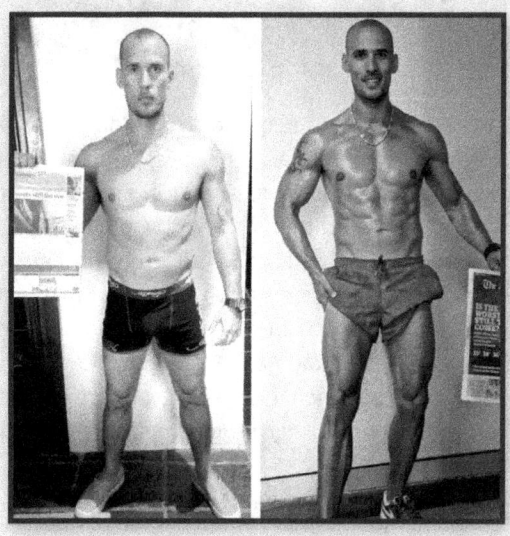

MATT

Matt was local to the area and heard about me through word of mouth and my Google reviews. His sleep patterns were poor and he was sick of feeling constantly tired. His body was ready for an overhaul and he was committed to getting that 6-pack!

I helped him create the structure he needed in a 12-week timeframe with the foundation of following the strict mindset, nutrition and training, which he needed.

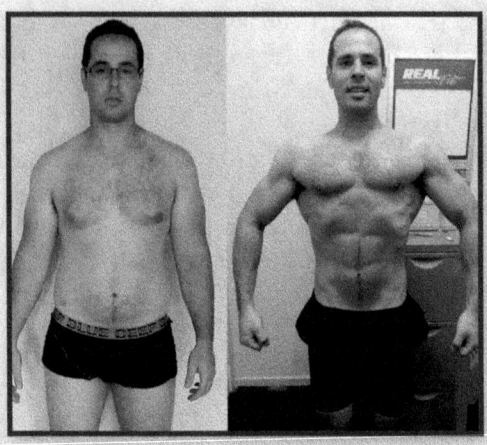

For Matt it wasn't so much about providing motivation, it was holding him accountable. As he says, "I knew if I let myself down, I would let Fred down as well. I like that we didn't use scales as a guide but rather fortnightly pictures to Fred to see my results. It was hard work but amazing and worth it. Like anything in life, you get out what you put in. I learnt how to obey the law of calories in versus calories out; also to live by the principle of food as 80% nutritional and 20% recreational. I have so much more energy. I have used the tools Fred gave me to keep up my fitness regime and for that I'm so grateful!

HOLLIE

With her own background in the fitness industry, Hollie was already fit and healthy but felt she had plateaued and was looking to push herself physically and mentally. She set a goal to be on stage in a fitness competition but found it daunting to get started. Hollie felt challenged by doubt, finding steady motivation, the level of commitment and time it required, as well as not knowing much about the competition industry itself.

Hollie's journey was unique in that she was already training a lot but she recognised she still had to make some significant lifestyle changes if she was going to step it up. She admits she loved going out and overindulging. My task was to help Hollie really focus her mindset to keep her goal always in her mind. I encouraged her to take a closer look at her nutrition and try to get in more of those early nights.

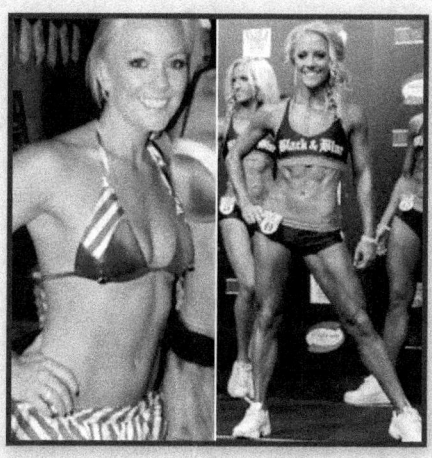

We worked together on the 3 pillars of Lean Muscle: nutrition, mindset and training. After 6 months of hard work, Hollie won one of the divisions in her competition and was runner-up in another. In Hollie's words, *"I am so grateful for Fred and his knowledge and motivation. He's taught me positive habits that will stick with me forever. I learnt preparation is key as well as discipline in learning how to ignore outside noise when you have a goal to achieve. Working with Fred has ensured that I will always be focused on my health. To this day my competition journey and being pregnant with my baby are my greatest physical achievements."*

RICHARD

Richard was looking to get more out of his general fitness routine that was keeping him in good shape but wasn't challenging him enough. He wanted to learn more, get on stage and hopefully win a physique title. He had heard I had a reputation for being a badass trainer but in a good way (thanks Richard ☺).

Richard didn't want to short cut anything so we set some challenges step by step over a 4 month period then evaluated if he was ready for a competition. Aiming high, Richard knew he would benefit from having someone like me to hold him accountable along the way to achieving his impressive results.

We didn't have to take the all or nothing approach, as Richard said, *"Fred moves you in a way that you're progressing each day, testing and measuring everything you do."* He came runner-up in a tough line-up on stage and was ecstatic to receive that trophy. Richard now instils so many great health and fitness habits in his new role as a father and being a role model to his son. Congratulations Richard!

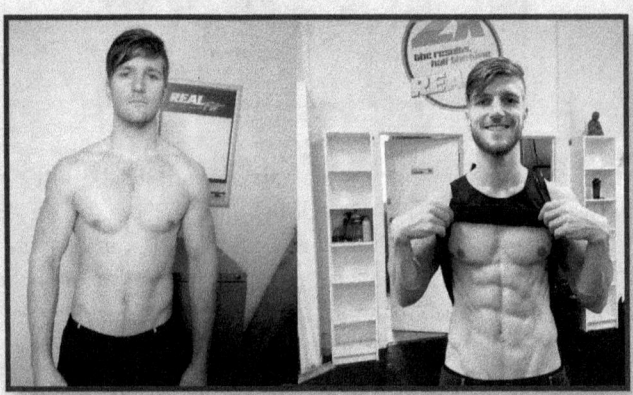

Check out Richard's abs in real time at leanmuscle.com. He's received thousands of views of him flexing his abs!

PETER

Peter worked in the corporate world and he had slowly begun overeating through the pressures of work. He'd put on weight, lost confidence and even putting on socks and doing up his shoelaces had become much harder than it used to be. He admits he did not understand the importance of eating right and thought just going to the gym meant everything would be fine.

I appeared just when he was ready to tackle his sliding lifestyle, initially in a 12-Week Challenge and then it extended beyond his expectations. Peter's biggest changes were nutrition, cutting out the alcohol and restructuring his training under my guidance. We added meditation and meal prep into his routine, which made a big difference. Realising that you can't out-train a bad diet, Peter became focused on cleaning up his food habits and started training "more sensibly" as he put it.

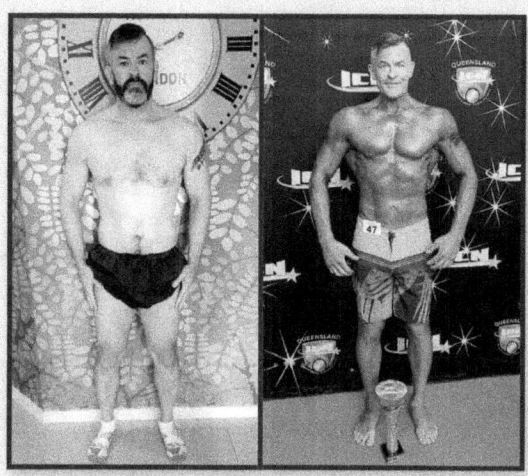

Peter kept a journal of everything and we shared regular communication and feedback on his meals and training. After 12 weeks Peter had dropped 15kgs and he felt great again. His body ached less and he said he had more energy than in his last year of high school many years ago! Peter's experience with the Lean Muscle program actually allowed him to find his true passion, as he left his corporate job to become a qualified Personal Trainer and accredited Sports Nutritionist!

He has also been competing very successfully in different fitness competitions and is training to compete in the Classic bodybuilder division in the Masters category. He is an amazing example to us all that age is just a number and it's never too late. Of our time working together Peter said, *"It's a personal investment that will reward you back tenfold."* I couldn't agree more. Check out Peter's video testimonial at leanmuscle.com.

CHAPTER 8

WORK WITH ME

A POST COVID-19 WORLD

Who would've thought a virus like this would stop the world in its tracks! Like countless others, it certainly had an enormous impact on my life and way of thinking. My studio was forced to shut during various periods of restrictions, affecting not only my livelihood, but also the livelihood of our trainers. When faced with a crisis, we can either sink or swim.

While I could have wallowed in all that I'd lost, COVID-19 graced us with a period to reflect and pivot to create a more sustainable business beyond bricks and mortar, and for that I'm grateful. I'm also fortunate to live in a lucky country. While Australia has not been immune to COVID-19, we have kept it under control.

I had always enjoyed training people online from time to time, and now I understood it was time to expand my previous dabbling. During COVID-19 I have created a membership site for the 12-Week

Challenge program, supported by a library of coaching and instructional videos for workouts at all levels and weekly group coaching.

While Realfit studio allows me to work one-on-one or with small groups, the 12-Week Challenge ignites my passion further by reaching individuals who have chosen their transformation through fitness and are no longer bound by the barrier of location. Here's to new beginnings!

THE 12-WEEK CHALLENGE

The 12-Week Challenge is a great barometer for change. Variations of the idea have been around since the mid '90s and been proven through and through by the early pioneers in the industry such as Bill Phillips. My own experience doing the 12-Week Challenge really enabled me to create the blueprint philosophy that I use to help my clients. I worked out my 'why', shifted my old beliefs, and enlisted a trainer to keep me accountable. This created a clear purpose for me each day of the Challenge to keep going, and keep going strong. Interested in being coached by me? Let's jump on a discovery call. Email me at info@leanmuscle.com with the subject line 'discovery call'.

The great thing about my 12-Week Challenge is its realistic time frame is designed to move you from maintenance to progression over the 12 weeks and you'll be amazed how much can be achieved in this period. It lifts you to a whole new level of living.

Here are my favourite reasons to embrace the 12-Week Challenge:
1. Never Boring – the change up of routine is important to stay accountable and this creates an exciting and dynamic feeling of not knowing what is ahead. Each day is different and engaging.
2. Results – you begin with the end in mind with clearly outlined goals. Often people become disheartened or intimidated by an overwhelming and narrow approach to exercise programs and routines that have no scope to enhance the individual's whole wellbeing. Nothing is learnt except how to lift a heavy weight or exercise mindlessly for a set time. This can lead to resigning

from their commitment early. My job is to wrap you up in the whole experience that keeps you excited to start each day's training and keeps you in the wellness zone all day. After all, most of the day is not spent training physically, but that time is so important in your mental preparation!
3. Guidelines – from mapping out what to eat, how to train and how to create a winner's mindset. It's a great way for those less experienced to follow a tried and tested system that works. I do that part of the program for you to simply follow.
4. Lifestyle – for busy parents to individuals, you can fit the program into a lunch break or when the little one is asleep, so when you make that commitment for 12 weeks of strict routine and healthy eating, you're far less likely to have that heavy feeling that you have a long workout to catch up on. It's manageable stages each day.

As a personal trainer it's my job to solve your problems when it comes to your fitness goals and, having had skin in the game for over four decades, I have collected and learnt from my fair share of challenges when it comes to helping clients ultimately reach their fitness goals.

The zero to hero journey is often fraught with friction when an individual takes on the challenge themselves. Remember even I needed a trainer when I undertook my own 12-Week Challenge to ensure that I would show up, shut up and follow a proven system. I have walked in your shoes and experienced your pain and ultimately many of your victories.

The challenge is tough and not for everyone so when I take on a potential client, the first thing we do is make sure we are the right fit for each other. The last thing I want to do is take your money and not have you commit to the 12-week journey.

Once you become a Lean Muscle graduate, you become part of the family. My formula for success is based on the two things I do really well, test and measure. This approach weeds out any past beliefs and provides a great feedback mechanism.

UNLOCKING MY 3 PROFICIENCIES

The Lean Muscle program is not just about gaining a six-pack (which no doubt you will achieve if that's your desire), it's a holistic body transformation where you get to feel better, look better and perform better. It's a system to change your strength and fitness levels and exceed your previous limits. And we achieve this with the following.

1. Efficiency of exercise

When working out on the Lean Muscle 12-Week Challenge program the goal is to get you stronger safely. Exercising for strength with the correct technique will help you expand your comfort zone, and when done well, will help lead you to your desired outcome.

2. Nutrition reform

The age old debate of 90% diet and 10% exercise doesn't hold true in my opinion unless you're a seasoned bodybuilder counting calories and meticulous with meal prep and manipulating carbs before a show. In reality I've found it's in favour of exercise, so I say it's 60% exercise and 40% diet. That doesn't mean you can gobble down anything in sight, it means if you have a more balanced view you'll be able to see the change that's needed, and you won't view food as the holy grail to transform your physique – you will view it the same as you view your training – do it often, and do it well.

3. Optimisation of your mind

If you look for limits, that is what you will find (and I promise you, you will find them), so expand your comfort zone until it envelops your limits.

The mind is often overlooked. I recall when I first started testing my mindfulness system with Lean Muscle graduates, listening daily to an audio recording and visualising their success, it greatly helped them gain clarity and focus on their goal, while keeping the gremlins and naysayers at bay.

Our mind is a powerful resource when we align it with our true self.

TRAIN SMART

Rather than look at a challenge as a short-term solution, fitness is a lifelong commitment, and it must start somewhere. Taking on a challenge, like my 12-Week Challenge will help you understand the work required to achieve long lasting results and to maintain a healthy body, mind and lifestyle.

Many believe only a selected number of people have what it takes to achieve great strength, hypertrophy, fat loss and cardiovascular conditioning simultaneously over a short amount of time like a 12 week period.

Well, let me tell you that YOU can, it IS possible and you do not need to take any synthetic drugs to help you get there. I'll show you how you can do it the natural way, using education, dedication and hard work to get you there. I can guarantee results because I am a master coach with over four decades of experience helping people achieve physical strength as well as aesthetic changes in just 12 weeks.

I know, this is a massive statement, but time and again I have seen that when my clients commit, they become accountable for their own wellbeing and harnessing these 'superpowers' which allows them to *really* shift and change their current reality. When you work with somebody as experienced as I am, besides physically changing your body, your mindset is upgraded which significantly impacts your life for the better. You can reach that place you've been imagining.

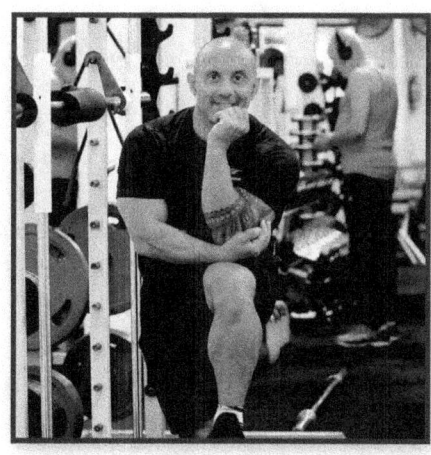

Time and time again I have witnessed how powerful this 12-Week Challenge is, with clients' results speaking for themselves. Word spread about these results so quickly that a large supplement company took an interest in my method and commissioned me to work with them. Together we helped thousands of people undergo transformations, developing strong relationships and changing their lives forever.

12 weeks is not a long time in the scheme of things, and 12 weeks is all you need to change your life for the better. You can reach your fitness goal in this challenge if you are motivated enough to begin and follow the guidelines as set out within the program. The program is mapped out for you, including what to eat and when, how to train, how to keep your mind sharp and how to stretch, improve and revisit your goals. Even if you are not as experienced as the next person, we start from wherever suits you and scale things up from there with guidance every step of the way.

I have developed and delivered some unprecedented body transformations in short periods of time over the past 30 years; every time, no matter the age, condition or genetics. I will stand by my promise that if you want it badly enough, I can make it happen for you. The Lean Muscle program is designed for you to safely and comfortably help you reach your goals with *Sweat Swear Smile* sprinkled in of course.

To help you understand more about the experience, I have answered the top 10 most asked questions below about the 12-Week Challenge.

> How can I join the program?

> Watch my webinar at leanmuscle.com and afterwards you will find a link to book a call with me to discuss any questions you may have, as well as to ensure we are a good fit for each other.

Do I need to go to a gym?

As mentioned earlier in this book, you can train wherever you want, if training at home make sure the environment you choose is dedicated for training. One of the things I have found is that if you are equipped with the 'right tools' you can work out anywhere at any time. You will require 'tools of the trade' which I will explain once you board the program.

How will you coach me?

One of the great things about being online is that no matter where you are in the world, if you have access to the Internet, you can be coached! My digital membership, mobile friendly coaching platform is continually evolving. Since the inception of our 12-week program, I have now developed other programs based on my clients' feedback. To know more, simply go to leanmuscle.com. You can check out Lean Muscle YouTube channel for sample videos by following the link at leanmuscle.com.

You will be supported by comprehensive written material and audio recordings constantly being tweaked using my own test and measure strategies. I continually request feedback from my graduates on how we can improve the program because there is always room for improvement!

What level of support will I get?

All 12-Week Challenge participants will receive a daily SMS and email as well as access to the Facebook Group #LeanMuscleEnthusiasts. You can search the group for past topics and questions, and if you have a question that's not been answered, I encourage you to post your question in the group where we will respond within a few hours. The group will also help keep you accountable.

Included are weekly group calls to discuss progress, go through what you're experiencing and answer any questions. These calls are recorded if you cannot participate live.

Will I do the challenge on my own or as part of a group?

The great thing about my online 12-Week Challenge is that it's done in your own time at your own pace. Even though you are doing the challenge on your own (whether in a home gym or at a gym), you never have to feel alone. I want to hear about your experiences and questions at every step.

> Will I need to take before and after pictures and share them?

I know not all of us are social creatures where we need to share everything through the web however my own research suggests as part of keeping you accountable I highly recommend you take 'before' and 'after' pictures for yourself. Our training modules will allow you to upload your 'before' picture however you do not have to share them if you do not want to and we totally respect your wishes. This is a purely personal choice. I have found when people have the picture to refer back to, it springboards them forwards and reminds them of why they made the commitment in the first place. They hold themselves accountable. The transformation is your personal journey and you are always in control whether you choose to share it or not

> What is the investment for a challenge like this?

A challenge like this is an investment in your future health and wellness. If you would like to know more, join the 12-Week Challenge Masterclass Webinar where I walk through what we cover, explain the level of commitment required, and we can then hop on a call and discuss the investment price including payment plan options

Do I need to take any supplements?

> No. If you wish to skyrocket your results, we often recommend a protein powder once you board the program.

What if I have an existing injury or cannot complete the challenge?

> Pre-existing injuries that require attention need to be checked by your health professional, especially when undergoing a 12-Week Challenge. I strongly recommend you get their approval before commencing any strenuous activity. We do not diagnose or treat injuries as outlined by the Terms & Conditions of the program on the website.
>
> In regards to stopping the challenge (perhaps life just got in the way), we don't offer any return on investment so please ensure the challenge is right for you before commencing. The last thing we want is to take your money with no commitment on your behalf!

> **What happens when I complete the 12-Week Challenge?**

You get to keep all the material you've gained along the way for life, so you can maintain the best version of you for the long-term. You become a Graduate of the Lean Muscle program and the virtual high-fives will pour in from me and your wider support group. My biggest wish is for you to take learnings here for life and pay it forward by sharing your success with others.

I believe everything has a start and finish. I want to have a lasting impression on your life. The program is designed to give you the knowledge to continue your fitness lifestyle beyond the program. If you miss us, would like continued support on the way to your end game, you can come back and redo the challenge – you're family now!

This program is suited for action takers and those open to learning. It's not for the faint hearted or those who want results with little or no effort. Regardless of your fitness level, you can become a graduate of the 12-Week Challenge, and be another raving fan inspiring others to take action in their fitness journey.

|||||

THE LEAN MUSCLE WAY WORKS

A big statement yes, but I can tell you, you don't need to be taking copious amounts of supplements and performance enhancing drugs. The key to my training is to expand your comfort zone until it swallows your previous limits, and you will always be in progression, not maintenance.

When the correct technique and momentum comes into play it will no doubt keep you out of pain and avoiding injuries. If you train your body and mind as not being a threat to yourself you will no doubt tap into your most primal energy levels: focus + power + convincing your inner superhero to come out!

WHY LISTEN TO ME?

Chances are you picked up this book because it resonated with you, whether intrigued by the title or you'd done your research on me and I'm grateful for the opportunity to connect with you. I trust the content gives you a better understanding of my values, and encompasses an understanding of how you should view fitness whatever age or level you are at. This book is about always seeking progress rather than perfection. You will become a better athlete if you focus on progress, putting your health at the forefront of your life.

Lean Muscle was founded for one simple reason – to create and execute the most effective health and fitness model in the online personal training space. This is where my passion bubbles over, and I am extremely dedicated and enthusiastic to bring you the best of my knowledge and experience, including remaining at the forefront of real world application to all aspects of physical conditioning. You want the lowdown on what I stand for, the why and how it benefits you.

At Lean Muscle we see it's easy to talk the talk, but to walk the walk is so much harder. I am arguably the most transparent personal trainer you'll meet and you can directly interact with me on any of my social media platforms.

As a personal trainer and studio owner (with a team of seven trainers), it is imperative I invest heavily in continued education. This requires constant dedication and commitment to be a lateral thinker and you will find I am informed and qualified in almost every aspect of the global fitness trends, and backed up by real world experience training real people to achieve often famous and sometimes notorious results!

I do not believe in standing back or feeding your ego with bullsh%#! In fact I like to *really* get stuck into every aspect of your life that you are prepared to open to me. No other way is appropriate for the level of commitment and investment you are making for your health.

IS ONLINE PT FOR ME?

Thanks to the Internet, there really are no more barriers to starting your new wellbeing path. You can create a dedicated space to work out anywhere to find that 'white-line fever'. We then cover every angle of health and fitness providing online videos, chats, forums, recipes, examples, photos, relatable explanations and common errors to look out for as well as vital support for those questions you have. No question is too small and you'll have access to so many other questions and answers that have already been asked by people starting out just like you.

The most common questions clients ask are to do with the level of accountability and their initial misperceptions around food and nutrition. This is why I created an active Facebook group with thousands of members and it's growing every day. It's a safe place for people that want to post real life questions, as we are all so supportive of each other's efforts and unique challenges. After all, we are all on the same journey – right? Check us out at facebook.com/groups/leanmuscleenthusiasts

So whenever you're not sure, you can drop us a line. On the accountability side, people often reach out to me and need some encouragement like this:

> Hi Fred, I'm enjoying the program, especially the 3 pillars of mind muscle and nutrition but to be honest I'm finding I lack the drive to do it myself ... help!

> Thanks for being honest and transparent. Have you revisited your goals and broken them up to small chunks? What have been your wins this week?

> Well, I made a deadline to stop eating by 7pm and I've been getting a good 8 hours sleep. I've been drinking a lot more water too. I even fasted for 24 hours – it wasn't too hard.

> Great! These are really important 'small wins' – remember to keep at it and these wins will increase over time, now that's a step in the right direction!

> Yes you're right, I'm feeling much better and I know I have to be patient with myself.

> Remember to also grade your workouts out of 10 in terms of effort. Check in on my Facebook group and post images and videos of your workout and what you're eating to keep yourself accountable. Also ask a family member to keep an eye on you, and trust me – you'd be surprised how much they can help you make changes.

> Great will do – thanks Fred! I so needed this chat, am feeling much better.

Or it might be something about nutrition like this question I received:

> Hi Fred, is this packet of spicy tomato lentil soup healthy?

> Check out the label carefully, do you recognise all of the ingredients?

> Not really Fred; what's vegetable concentrate?

> That's a sneaky way of saying salt.

> So are any packaged foods healthy Fred?

> Not in a real health and fitness lifestyle. Stick to natural foods that come from nature not a factory!

INGREDIENTS
VEGETABLE CONCENTRATE, THAI MINT, SUNFLOWER OIL, CUMIN (0.08%), BLACK PEPPER, CHILLI (0.02%).

May contain traces of egg, fish and crustacea

NUTRITIONAL INFORMATION

Servings per package: 2
Serving size: 250g

	Avg Quantity per Seving	Avg. Quantity per 100g
Energy	333kJ (80 Cal)	133kJ (32 Cal)
Protein	5.0 g	1.8 g
– gluten	0.0 g	0.0 g
Fat, total	1.0 g	0.6 g
– saturated	0.3 g	0.1 g
Carbohydrate	10.0 g	4.0 g
– sugars	3.0 g	1.1 g
Dietary fibre	4.0 g	1.4 g
Sodium	573 mg	229 mg

ARE WE THE RIGHT FIT?

I invite you to look beyond the ads of impressive six packs or perky glutes on social media and you'll find a cookie cutter approach that works for a small percentage of those who buy it, whose determination outweighs the distractions around them. Without interaction and accountability, it's far too easy to lose sight of your goal and stop altogether.

At Lean Muscle we get that you need a trusted and accountable personal trainer to cut through all the crap and confusion and get you long term results fast, while teaching you skills so you are empowered to continue your lifeline fitness journey beyond the program. We help you tailor your program to your goals and do not believe in leaving anything to chance!

For over four decades I've trained people from all walks of life, from elite athletes to celebrities, everyday folk, corporate and blue collar workers, strippers, and even a priest, but the one thing that holds true is everyone comes with a desire to change their life for the better. Through a conversation about each client's goals, abilities and level of commitment, I'm able to tailor each person's program so they can achieve their desired goal at a pace that works for them. It is through monitoring their nutrition plans, exercise review and measurements that we are able to progress.

Let's connect! leanmuscle.com

Don't forget you can also find me at my Realfit studio located in East Malvern, Victoria. I live and breathe fitness and everything I learn from my face-to-face clients goes towards helping my online family as well. Realfit studio is one of the highest Google-rated five star 'Gyms & Personal Trainers' in Australia since 2006.

CHAPTER 9

CONCLUSION

STAY COMMITTED TO YOUR GOALS

From what I have seen over the years, when people do not quickly see the results they want, they get frustrated and lose sight of the end game. Ditch the instant gratification because results simply do not happen overnight.

Never quit or give up on YOU, and that will give you the strength to play the long game. You can change your goals, but remain dedicated to you. Taking action day after day builds the foundation brick by brick and prevents you from sliding backwards and undoing your hard work. Know you will only see small changes to begin with, but use a tape measure and the fit of your clothes as your guide.

The purpose of this book is to also teach you life-long principles. If you are serious about making fitness a regular part of your life, you need to reinforce these foundations by replacing habits that don't support your dreams with ones that do, such as a healthy lifestyle change.

If you want to develop strength and get a lean muscular body, it takes hours in the gym—not just a few hours here and there, but hours on a consistent basis. You need to pursue your goal by getting into the gym day in and day out. Just like you make it a habit to brush your teeth or watch television before bed, incorporate that habit of getting to the gym.

Working out does not require as much effort as you think. The key is to really make time for what is important in your life. Not only will training change your physiological appearance, but also it will provide you with the mental tools necessary to succeed in anything you do (i.e. finances, business, and education).

IF YOU FAIL TO PLAN, YOU PLAN TO FAIL

Keep your eyes on the prize, prepare in advance and limit distractions.

What makes my clients so successful is that they create a schedule every single day so they can be more productive. We work on solidifying their daily objectives which makes them much more likely to stick to their list. At the end of the day it allows them to reflect on their day and be proud of hitting the accomplishments they set out.

Each night, before I go to sleep, I gaze at the ceiling and look back on the events of my day. When I achieve a lot throughout the day, I have a sense of accomplishment, a wonderful feeling that is infectious. The more tasks I complete throughout the day, the prouder I become. I notice the more demanding and daunting the task I complete, the more accomplished I feel. Of course, there are other days when I truly regret my lack of effort. When I fail to perform I am disappointed in myself that I've 'wasted' time. I wish I could go back and re-live that day so much more productively!

I have noticed throughout my life that people need motivation to engage themselves, whether it is internal, external, or subconscious, motivation is needed in order for an individual to act. People need to be pulled towards a vision. Sometimes it's hard to muster the motivation, but a written schedule and plan propels us to accomplish things – written words on paper solidify our efforts. This plan of action stimulates us to work hard and complete the schedule, especially if there is a sense of urgency.

I challenge you to write down a goal and a deadline for achieving that goal. Then chunk it down into smaller goals, and list weekly and daily actions you will take to achieve it. Be specific. Make it easy otherwise the battlefield of your thoughts will kick in and sabotage your efforts. Take a look below:

EXAMPLE OF PLANNING YOUR DAY

6:00 am – 6:30 am	Meditation
6:30 am – 7:30 am	Workout
7:30 am – 8:15 am	Shower, breakfast, revisit goals daily
8:15 am – 9:00 am	Travel/prepare for work
9:00 am – 5:00 pm	Work
5:00 pm – 6:00 pm	Travel/unwind from work
6:00 pm – 6:30 pm	Prepare tomorrow's training program (lists exercises and reps), reflect on today
6:30 pm – 7:30 pm	Dinner, meals for the next day ready to go
7:30 pm – 9:00 pm	Free time
9:00 pm – 9:30 pm	Write down goals for next day, prepare for sleep
9:30 pm	Lights out!

Another fabulous benefit of the 12-Week Challenge is it's perfect for anyone's schedule. You can do Week 1 at 3 o'clock in the morning if that works for you. The sample schedule is to emphasise the importance that training, mindset and nutrition must be solidified as part of your set routine. Everyone in the household can know and understand what your responsibility is to yourself and what you'll be doing at a set time.

A HEALTHY LAUGH

In the words of the late great comedian John Pinette:

> *"I have gotten a trainer.*
> *I went to the gym and I saw him and*
> *he said 'Give me a sit up,'*
> *and I said 'Oh nay, nay'.*
> *I go 'I don't do ups:*
> *sit ups, push ups, pull ups.*
> *I do do downs. I will sit down,*
> *I will lay down.*
> *Blackjack I'll double down.*
> *Give me a cheeseburger,*
> *I'll wolf that down.*
> *But no ups. Ups defy gravity,*
> *that's a law, I obey the law."*[1]

My passion for personal training is very evident through this book and my enthusiasm comes through strongly when I work with people to help them achieve their goals and really feel confident and happy in their own skin. If you have read to this point, I commend you for taking action to educate yourself.

I encourage you to be brutally honest with yourself and reflect on your journey thus far – what's working for you, what's not working, and whether NOW is the time to up your game? As you will have discovered, there is a minefield of information out there and it's easy to get lost and fail to take action.

I am the trainer who will be able to help you attain your perfect body with the right nutrition and exercise plan tailored to you, shifting and empowering your mindset, alongside your dedication and discipline to make that happen.

I know that we are all human and sometimes we can fall off the wagon. It is crucial to understand this is okay and to pick yourself up, dust yourself off, and get back on again.

AGEING GRACEFULLY

There are lots of so-called secrets to longevity and maintaining a healthy older age. I think you know me well enough by now to guess that my tips are very simple. Just as Mum taught me growing up, being positive and not sweating the small stuff is really important. Nowadays the physical effects of stress have become well-known facts. Meditation and a strong mindset help you handle those challenging situations in life, so you don't internalise the stress.

Having a goal to work towards in life keeps you motivated, full of purpose and keeps that spark in your eye, it doesn't have to be a fitness goal, whatever you are passionate about. Something as simple as being grateful for your family and friends each day can provide a great support for you to be courageous and follow that dream.

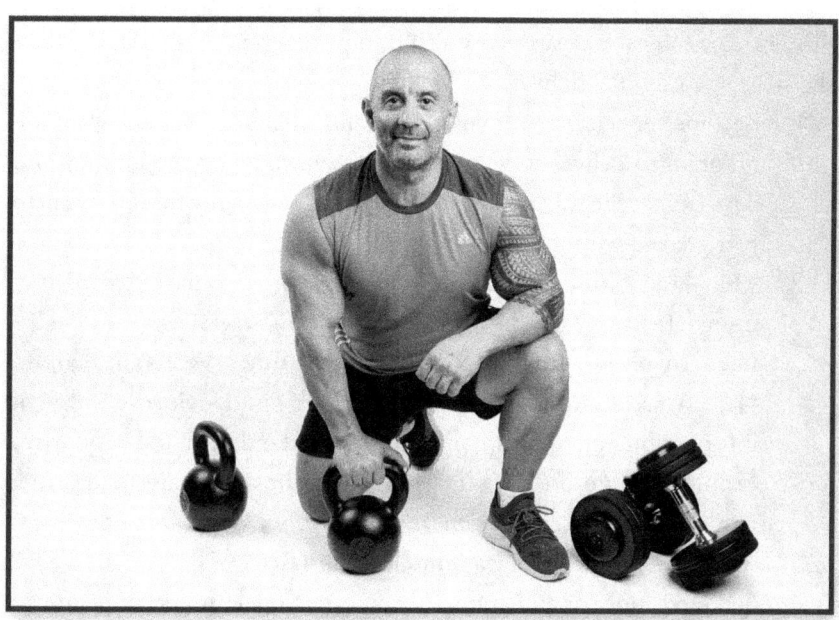

Another simple 'secret' to ageing gracefully is to eat as close to nature as possible. Think back to before the onslaught of processed food, ask yourself could your grandparents have eaten it? In most cases the answer is no, so stick with real food that has been part of a healthy diet for generations. Remember don't over consume, another by-product of the modern world and really detrimental to our health.

A final and somewhat harsh truth is that drinking alcohol speeds up the aging process. It makes you age, put on weight and makes your body acidic. Perhaps a glass of vino rosso to celebrate something special, but generally, I suggest keeping alcohol to a minimum so you can celebrate many more milestones.

YOUR INVITATION

If I was a betting man right now my guess is you are probably feeling like you have been drinking from a fire hose, and I totally get that overwhelm. The concepts I have outlined have taken me many decades to formulate (through that good old testing and measuring technique).

I wish I had something like this when I got started because I know it's not easy to power past those speed bumps that pop up in life. Here are the steps you can take right now:

1. Become very clear about your 'why' and what outcome you want the program to deliver to you, as I want you to enjoy the journey and have fun on the way (remember the *Smile* part in my title). I can help you prepare your 'how'.
2. Visit Lean Muscle YouTube channel where I have recorded a tonne of videos explaining how to do specific exercises
3. Get involved and hang out in my Facebook group #LeanMuscleEnthusiasts where you'll find videos full of information and a great community of like-minded and supportive people who are on the same mission to be a healthier and leaner version of themselves. You may find your support buddy here (facebook.com/groups/leanmuscleenthusiasts).
4. See food more as nutritional than recreational, and know you can have a balance by remembering the 80/20 rule.
5. Meditation has really changed my life, so get up earlier, sit in silence, acknowledge your day ahead and just let go; the universe has bigger plans for us all!
6. Do not see resistance training as a chore; instead see it as a reward for your body. We know the science is there to back it up and

think of how great you feel after a work out and how it sets up your day for positivity and productivity.
7. Be a belief system detective – test and measure before fobbing an idea off. Have an open and curious mind, and that invincible force will propel you to success.
8. Know that real change begins with YOU and your 'why'. Your message can also change other people's lives, so own it, use it, and share it. You just might empower someone else who will pay it forward too.
9. I invite you to check out my website at leanmuscle.com and complete your why before putting it on your fridge or your bathroom mirror (wherever you can see it daily) to revisit your goals every day for motivation.
10. Know I'm here for you – if you have a question connect with me on the LeanMuscleEnthusiasts Facebook Group or leanmuscle.com where your question asked not only helps you, but another on their fitness journey.

SPECIAL THANKS TO SOME VERY SPECIAL PEOPLE
(ACKNOWLEDGEMENTS)

I was beyond excited when Matt Preston provided a foreword to my book. I have come to know Matt through the studio and we have had a rewarding and memorable training experience together. Our philosophies meshed perfectly, and we learnt a lot from each other. Be sure to check out his book *More*, some truly delicious recipes starring vegetables that have more of everything: more flavour, more texture, more colour. Thanks for your support Matt!

IIIII

This book would not be complete without mentioning my mum. She is a wonderful example of what it means not to allow age to define you, and that your attitude determines your altitude! At the time of writing this book, she is 90 years young and she continues to inspire and motivate me every day.

As Mum's 'unofficial' personal trainer, when I go visit we don't just eat her favourite minestrone soup, I make sure she trains! It could be something as simple as a toe touch or hip thrusts, followed with a foam roller stretch and then on her stationary bike for 30 minutes – that's where you'll find her every day at 3pm. Did you know she also stars in my videos? I have clients of all ages.

My mum taught me to keep a positive spirit and leading by example, especially during tougher times she was and still is, inspiring. Always showing courage, and reminding us all of the importance of staying connected to family. No matter where my path took me, I knew I always had my mum to lean on.

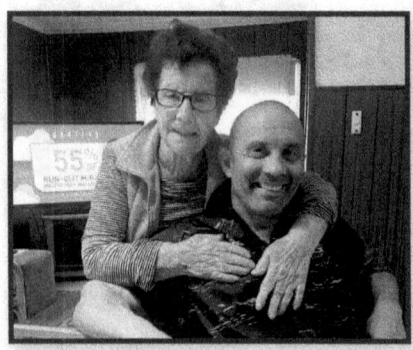 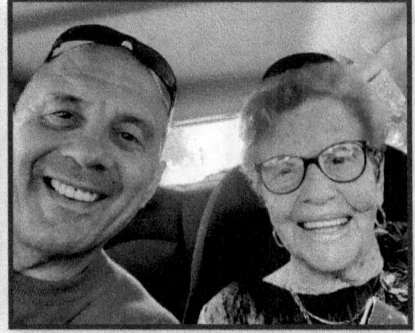

As far back as I can remember my mum was fearless, always willing to try new things and venture into unknown territory. She was never one to hold a grudge or play the victim, and always looked to create a better future, making brave changes and teaching us the importance of quality in life. Always enthusiastic, never hesitating to be her best and show us that it is important to aim for what we want in life, but also that we must try again if we fail.

I don't think I would have had the courage to pursue my dreams without my mum's strength and support throughout my life. I'd also

ACKNOWLEDGEMENTS

like to pay homage to my dearly departed father who provided me with everything I need in my life through his love, support and wisdom. To this day I have never meet a more gentle soul and wiser man. You live in my heart every day and I'll never forget the words of wisdom you offered in all parts of my life whether it was about sport, fitness, my career or everyday situations. You listened and then gave great advice – thank you Pa.

|||||

Thank you to my brother Tony for setting the standard, and boy did he set it high, winning every imaginable medal at the 3 grades of VFL/AFL Football. He was a trailblazer, never quitting. Between 1986 and 2002 Tony played 283 senior games and kicked 95 goals. He was well loved at the Western Oval, and throughout the 1990s was one of the most readily identifiable figures in football. His son Thomas has now led the way winning best and fairest in the AFL Premiership Flag in 2016. What a legacy.

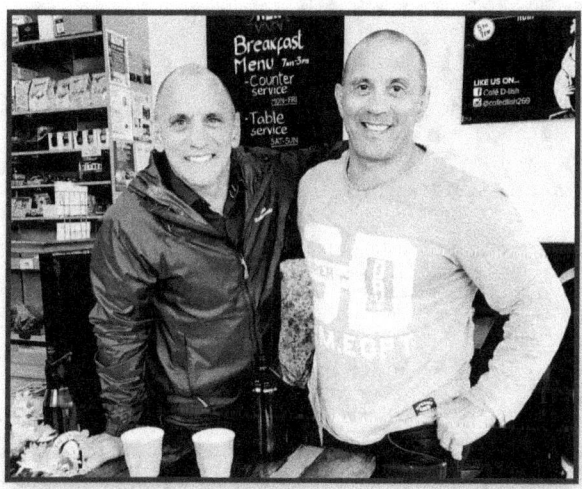

Tony was my steadfast supporter and a great partner in crime growing up. Seeing Tony's determination helped me develop my own. I knew if I could match Tony's willpower, I could achieve anything.

|||||

Thank you to my sister Linda, for always being a great sounding board and always being there for me, no matter what. Getting her female perspective on life led me to make some great decisions, so thanks Sis!

If it were not for my older brother John's observation of my interest in the sport of bodybuilding, I probably would have had to take another direction altogether. I'll be ever grateful to him for my first handmade concrete barbell, and for gifting me my first gym membership. Thank you Bro.

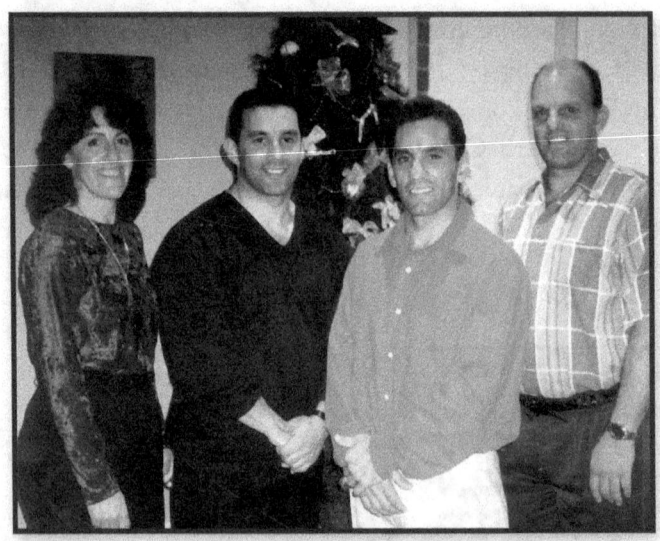

|||||

This book aims to be so much more than words on paper. Something that ignites a spark, to be the catalyst for people that have had something holding them back, to finally rid themselves of their old obstacles. The old cliché holds true that if you don't move it you will lose it, and hopefully many people can be empowered to heed those words so they live a long, happy life.

A WORTHY CAUSE

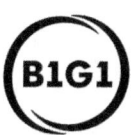
Your purchase of this book also supported a worthy cause. I am on a mission to serve and help create a world full of giving that benefits everyone. I partnered up with 'B1G1' Business for Good (Buy1Give1), which is a non-profit organisation with a mission to create a world that is full of giving.

B1G1 specifically helps small and medium-size businesses achieve more social impact by embedding giving activities into everyday business operations. Know that when you purchase this book or any of my services, a portion goes to charity to help fund education, environment, food, health, shelter, income generation (skills and training, supporting local entrepreneurship and business training), human rights and life enhancement programs across the globe.

OVER TO YOU

I have spent over 18 months writing and rewriting my book with the help of my publisher because I wanted it to be a book full of advice that propels you into action. There is only so much I can share in a book because each and every person is unique (with their own body and mindset challenges to overcome), so it cannot replace working directly with you to achieve your fitness goals.

I encourage you to read the book again to grasp the concepts, and help you take your fitness understanding to the next level. And when you're ready, I invite you to get on a complimentary discovery call. Email me at info@leanmuscle.com with the subject line 'discovery call'.

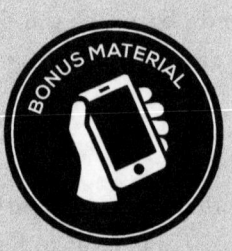

Fred is sharing bonus material.

In order to receive this, simply email him at info@leanmuscle.com.

ABOUT THE AUTHOR

With over four decades in the fitness industry, Fred Liberatore's knowledge and experience has created one passionate and highly sought-after Master Coach and Body Transformation Expert! From the moment he stepped into a gym as a young teenager, Fred was hooked on learning about health, nutrition and fitness. Fred's unique commitment to testing and measuring the countless techniques and fads that have come and gone over his fitness career, has empowered truly incredible results for himself and hundreds of his clients.

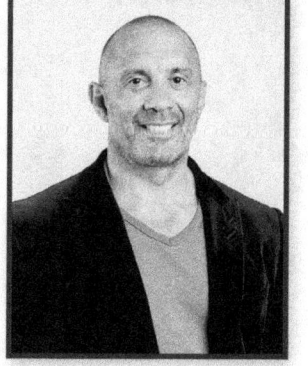

Fred knows what works and what doesn't, so he can tailor training programs to everyone's unique body type, needs and personal goals. Fred has the edge over 99% of personal trainers, coaches and health experts because he understands the physical aspect of training and nutrition in the finest detail. Importantly Fred also combines this with the mental edge he has discovered after years of studying the world's top peak performance experts.

Fred's philosophy has always been to train hard, no excuses. His own peak fitness is a reflection of that winning numerous bodybuilding titles, which culminated in the coveted title of Mr Australia in the NABBA Masters in 2000. Fred went on to also win the NABBA Grand Master title in 2016.

Fred has stood the test of time, with over four decades in the fitness industry. He loves empowering people to achieve physical success, no matter what their goals are.

Supported by his devoted family and friends, Fred has since sold his RealFit gym in Melbourne and is now a keynote speaker, travelling the world and delivering valuable content to organisations, ensuring his legacy lives on. He is also an online coach.

Fred's lifelong goal is simple: to create a holistic approach to health, nutrition and anti-aging that inspires fulfilment in all aspects of life for his clients.

NOTE FROM AUTHOR:

Congratulations! As a reader of my book, you have now qualified to get together with me on a one-to-one discovery call. Together, let's discuss your goals. All you need to do is contact me at info@leanmuscle.com with the subject line 'discovery call'. I look forward to speaking with you.

ENDNOTES

INTRODUCTION
1   The Victorian Football League (VFL) expanded to become the Australian Football League (AFL) in 1990

CHAPTER 1: THE BIRTH OF REALFIT
1   Grucza, R., Lecroart, J.L., Hauser, J.J. et al. Dynamics of sweating in men and women during passive heating. *Europ. J. Appl. Physiol.* 54, 309–314 (1985). https://doi.org/10.1007/BF00426151 and Kaciuba-Uscilko H, Grucza R. Gender differences in thermoregulation. *Current Opinion in Clinical Nutrition and Metabolic Care.* 2001 Nov;4(6):533-536. DOI: 10.1097/00075197-200111000-00012

2   Keele University. "Swearing Can Actually Increase Pain Tolerance." ScienceDaily. ScienceDaily, 13 July 2009. www.sciencedaily.com/releases/2009/07/090713085453.htm

3   Noel E. Brick, Megan J. McElhinney, Richard S. Metcalfe, 'The effects of facial expression and relaxation cues on movement economy, physiological, and perceptual responses during running.' *Psychology*

of Sport and Exercise, Volume 34, 2018, https://doi.org/10.1016/j.psychsport.2017.09.009

CHAPTER 3: BODY

1. George E, Deakin University, 'What you need to know about gut health', online article, accessed Feb 18, 2021. https://this.deakin.edu.au/self-improvement/what-you-need-to-know-about-gut-health

2. Clapp, M., Aurora, N., Herrera, L., Bhatia, M., Wilen, E., & Wakefield, S. (2017). 'Gut microbiota's effect on mental health: The gut-brain axis'. *Clinics and practice*, 7(4), 987. https://doi.org/10.4081/cp.2017.987
Zhang, Y. J., Li, S., Gan, R. Y., Zhou, T., Xu, D. P., & Li, H. B. (2015). 'Impacts of gut bacteria on human health and diseases'. *International journal of molecular sciences*, 16(4), 7493–7519. https://doi.org/10.3390/ijms16047493

3. St-Onge, M. P., & Gallagher, D. (2010). 'Body composition changes with aging: the cause or the result of alterations in metabolic rate and macronutrient oxidation?'. *Nutrition* (Burbank, Los Angeles County, Calif.), 26(2), 152–155. https://doi.org/10.1016/j.nut.2009.07.004

4. Better Health Channel, 'Metabolic Syndrome', Victorian Government, accessed February 17, https://www.betterhealth.vic.gov.au/health/conditionsandtreatments/metabolic-syndrome

5. Trexler, E. T., Smith-Ryan, A. E., & Norton, L. E. (2014). 'Metabolic adaptation to weight loss: implications for the athlete'. *Journal of the International Society of Sports Nutrition*, 11(1), 7. https://doi.org/10.1186/1550-2783-11-7

6. Breslau, N., Roth, T., Rosenthal, L., & Andreski, P. (1996). 'Sleep disturbance and psychiatric disorders: a longitudinal epidemiological study of young adults.' *Biological psychiatry*, 39(6), 411–418. https://doi.org/10.1016/0006-3223(95)00188-3

7. Pigeon, W.R., Bishop, T.M. & Krueger, K.M. 'Insomnia as a Precipitating Factor in New Onset Mental Illness: a Systematic Review of Recent Finding's. *Curr Psychiatry* Rep 19, 44 (2017). https://doi.org/10.1007/s11920-017-0802-x

8   University of Chicago, 'Investigations: Sleep away Fat?', University of Chicago Magazine. accessed February 17 2021. http://magazine.uchicago.edu/0010/research/invest-sleep.htm

9   Hirotsu, C., Tufik, S., & Andersen, M. L. (2015).' Interactions between sleep, stress, and metabolism: From physiological to pathological conditions'. *Sleep science* (Sao Paulo, Brazil), 8(3), 143–152. https://doi.org/10.1016/j.slsci.2015.09.002

10 Nedeltcheva, A. V., Kilkus, J. M., Imperial, J., Schoeller, D. A., & Penev, P. D. (2010). 'Insufficient sleep undermines dietary efforts to reduce adiposity'. *Annals of internal medicine*, 153(7), 435–441. https://doi.org/10.7326/0003-4819-153-7-201010050-00006

11 Okamoto-Mizuno, K., & Mizuno, K. (2012). 'Effects of thermal environment on sleep and circadian rhythm'. *Journal of physiological anthropology*, 31(1), 14. https://doi.org/10.1186/1880-6805-31-14

12 Bernert RA, Turvey CL, Conwell Y, Joiner TE. 'Association of Poor Subjective Sleep Quality With Risk for Death by Suicide During a 10-Year Period: A Longitudinal, Population-Based Study of Late Life'. *JAMA Psychiatry.* 2014;71(10):1129–1137. doi:10.1001/jamapsychiatry.2014.1126

13 Lee, P., Smith, S., Linderman, J., Courville, A. B., Brychta, R. J., Dieckmann, W., Werner, C. D., Chen, K. Y., & Celi, F. S. (2014). 'Temperature-acclimated brown adipose tissue modulates insulin sensitivity in humans'. *Diabetes*, 63(11), 3686–3698. https://doi.org/10.2337/db14-0513

14 Rafalson, L., Donahue, R. P., Stranges, S., Lamonte, M. J., Dmochowski, J., Dorn, J., & Trevisan, M. (2010). 'Short sleep duration is associated with the development of impaired fasting glucose: the Western New York Health Study'. *Annals of epidemiology*, 20(12), 883–889.

15 Lidia Mínguez-Alarcón, Audrey J Gaskins, Yu-Han Chiu, Carmen Messerlian, Paige L Williams, Jennifer B Ford, Irene Souter, Russ Hauser, Jorge E Chavarro, 'Type of underwear worn and markers of testicular function among men attending a fertility center', *Human*

Reproduction, Volume 33, Issue 9, September 2018, Pages 1749–1756, https://doi.org/10.1093/humrep/dey259

16 West, K. 'Naked and Unashamed: Investigations and Applications of the Effects of Naturist Activities on Body Image, Self-Esteem, and Life Satisfaction'. *J Happiness Stud* 19, 677–697 (2018). https://doi.org/10.1007/s10902-017-9846-1

17 Uvnäs-Moberg, K., Handlin, L., & Petersson, M. (2015). 'Self-soothing behaviors with particular reference to oxytocin release induced by non-noxious sensory stimulation'. *Frontiers in psychology*, 5, 1529. https://doi.org/10.3389/fpsyg.2014.01529

CHAPTER 4: NUTRITION

1 Catherine Chin-Chance, Kenneth S. Polonsky, Dale A. Schoeller, 'Twenty-Four-Hour Leptin Levels Respond to Cumulative Short-Term Energy Imbalance and Predict Subsequent Intake', *The Journal of Clinical Endocrinology & Metabolism*, Volume 85, Issue 8, 1 August 2000, Pages 2685–2691, https://doi.org/10.1210/jcem.85.8.6755

2 Parr EB, Camera DM, Areta JL, Burke LM, Phillips SM, Hawley JA, et al. (2014) 'Alcohol Ingestion Impairs Maximal Post-Exercise Rates of Myofibrillar Protein Synthesis following a Single Bout of Concurrent Training'. *PLoS ONE* 9(2): e88384. https://doi.org/10.1371/journal.pone.0088384

CHAPTER 5: EXERCISES

1 Pedro A. Latorre-Román, Felipe García-Pinillos, Víctor M. Soto-Hermoso, Marcos Muñoz-Jiménez. 'Effects of 12 weeks of barefoot running on foot strike patterns, inversion–eversion and foot rotation in long-distance runners'. *Journal of Sport and Health Science*, 2016; DOI: 10.1016/j.jshs.2016.01.004

2 The Department of Health, (April 12 2019) 'Australia's Physical Activity and Sedentary Behaviour Guidelines and the Australian 24-Hour Movement Guidelines', Australian Government Department of Health, accessed February 17 2021 https://www1.health.gov.au/

internet/main/publishing.nsf/Content/health-pubhlth-strateg-phys-act-guidelines#npa1864

3   Johannsmeyer, S., Candow, D. G., Brahms, C. M., Michel, D., & Zello, G. A. (2016). 'Effect of creatine supplementation and drop-set resistance training in untrained aging adults'. *Experimental gerontology*, 83, 112–119. https://doi.org/10.1016/j.exger.2016.08.005

4   Fink, J., Schoenfeld, B. J., Kikuchi, N., & Nakazato, K. (2018). 'Effects of drop set resistance training on acute stress indicators and long-term muscle hypertrophy and strength'. *The Journal of sports medicine and physical fitness*, 58(5), 597–605. https://doi.org/10.23736/S0022-4707.17.06838-4

CONCLUSION

1   Pinette, John. (20 November 2014) 'I'm starving – the gym'. Comedy Station, accessed via YouTube February 17, 2021, https://www.youtube.com/watch?v=O7xyO91dizQ

SWEAT SWEAR SMILE

FRED'S TIPS

Day 1	Thanks for joining the Lean Muscle program; super excited to have you on-board! We'll be supporting you with daily tips to keep you grounded in the principles of success; no excuses. Take a 'before' shot if you'd like a physical comparison to look back on in 12 weeks.
Day 2	Today is the second day of the rest of your new, improved life looking and feeling better than ever! Congratulations on making this commitment.
Day 3	Your goal is not a single desire that can be granted in an instant. Never forget it's a gradual process that takes time and commitment to the work that needs to be done each week, each day and each moment.
Day 4	Sleep is your superpower. Make it a ritual to go to bed early and rise early at the same time each morning. Your body loves routine.
Day 5	Before you eat something remember that body fat is the result of eating processed foods and refined carbohydrates. Stick to natural food.
Day 6	Be sure to win the nightly battle against cravings. Have a drink of water instead and hit the sack to resist temptation.

Day 7	Well done on the last day of your first week, momentum builds from here as you take it all in, understanding the requirements of your body type. Be sure to check the online training and mark it as complete.
Day 8	Put a hold on, or better yet, a stop to alcohol consumption. It's counterproductive on a health and fitness journey, those drunk 'munchies' can undermine all your efforts.
Day 9	Don't forget to do your homework on your nutrition and keep a journal to really elevate your learning and empower your convictions from deep within.
Day 10	A true body transformation is a balance between attitude, diet and exercise. The first two will sustain you as you exercise.
Day 11	Welcome new ideas to help you think differently so you can break out from your old mindset, your old beliefs and unhelpful behaviours.
Day 12	Eat for fuel; not taste. This is easy to mistake but be critical in your reasoning behind your choices and you will marvel at the difference it makes in the mirror.

Day 13	Just as you prepare physically for your workouts with the right clothing, equipment and location, don't neglect your mental preparation. Keep those motivational words running on repeat throughout the day and as you work out.
Day 14	Remember it's not about the weight; it's about the contraction. It will take your physique to a new level.
Day 15	Jump into the benefits of meditation. It's not something to be mastered; rather it is an anchor for the mind amid the daily hustle. Daily practice keeps us centred and focused.
Day 16	Did you know that your body treats calories differently when you exercise? The calories you eat go towards refuelling your body; giving you another reason to move.
Day 17	Remember to maintain natural breathing during meditation. Don't overthink it or you'll unconsciously alter it, which means your mind is busy thinking rather connecting to the universe.
Day 18	Re-establish your game plan and stay focused. Ignore advice and opinions that do not support your goal.
Day 19	Ditch your trigger foods. They belong in your past and no longer serve you.

Day 20	Building a good meditation habit requires effort and consistency. It's like working out; the more you do it the better the rewards become.
Day 21	Eggs are just about the best source of protein you can get, containing 8 amino acids for muscle growth and recovery.
Day 22	Get comfortable with discomfort. Breaking old, negative thought patterns is difficult, the brain likes familiar thoughts but over time the mind will adjust and want to avoid those dead end thoughts in favour of the new opportunities opening up through 'discomfort'.
Day 23	Did you know that capsicums have tremendous benefits and are an excellent source of Vitamin C and A? They are also great for lung health.
Day 24	Remember portion control at every meal; use the palm/fist/thumb rule to easily measure protein, carbs and fat intake.
Day 25	Start your day with meditation. Getting up earlier in the quiet of dawn connects you to a higher level of focus and dedication.
Day 26	Ensure you eat within 30 minutes of your workout in order to promote weight loss and lean muscle (check out the video on post-workout meals at leanmuscle.com).

Day 27	Did you find a 'buddy' to help keep you in check and hold you accountable to your goal? How are they doing? Is there something to improve on?
Day 28	Go bananas – they are high in Vitamin B6 and help to maintain a healthy nervous system.
Day 29	Don't stress the small stuff, keep things in perspective and remember this goal is something you've been dreaming of so your new schedule is non-negotiable.
Day 30	Fasting is the most effective way to reduce calorie intake; it restores a balance between fed and fasted metabolism.
Day 31	You can eat as many natural, raw fruits and vegetables as you want without any negative impact on your physique.
Day 32	Remember at first the signs of progress are subtle, you might be doing everything right and still think nothing is happening, but let me assure it is. Internal changes and readjustments are happening that will manifest externally in their own time. You want these changes to be long-term so short-cuts don't work.

Day 33	"If you ain't cheating you ain't trying." This expression reminds us we are human and allowed to make mistakes without actually falling off the wagon. Just be sure not to overdo it. Check out our video on cheat meals at leanmuscle.com.
Day 34	Be sure to use only extra virgin olive oil. It is the purest with more antioxidants as well as being the tastiest.
Day 35	Did you know that the glycaemic index is a measurement that gauges the speed at which sugars in food are released into the blood stream? It pays to understand where your food sits on the index.
Day 36	Have you tried adding seaweed or kelp to your diet? It's a great marine plant with iodine and alkali which helps to heal your cuts and grazes, and it's great for your metabolism and body overall.
Day 37	Fasting helps to regulate the hormones in your body so that you experience true hunger in its primal form.
Day 38	Schedule your training sessions into your diary the same as an appointment. Training is non-negotiable, just like that meeting with your boss.
Day 39	Stretching helps improve your range of motion, which is said to also slow the degeneration of your joints.

Day 40	Whole and rolled oats are one of the richest sources of inositol, which assists the proper metabolism of fats.
Day 41	Swearing during exercise can improve performance and even help you deal with pain so get f&#king swearing (in the right place).
Day 42	Sugar feeds bacteria and interferes with vitamin C, be sure to read labels and don't consume products with more than 10g sugar per 100g serve.
Day 43	Almonds are one of the richest sources of vitamin E, which is essential for heart and muscle vitality and blood circulation.
Day 44	When you are sweating mother nature is working for you as sweat is a detoxifying agent and is great for your skin.
Day 45	Stretching prior to exercise allows your muscles to loosen up and become better able to withstand the impact of the activity you choose to do.
Day 46	Fasting has been shown to improve brain function as it increases the production of an important protein called 'brain-derived neurotrophic factor', which promotes learning and memory which are vital for a longer, healthier and happier life.

Day 47	If you look after your body for the first 50 years, it will look after you for the next 50.
Day 48	To get the best results from your fitness schedule, allow your body enough time to recover and repair, this can vary between individuals.
Day 49	Stand proud in everything you do. 'Your attitude determines your altitude' – Zig Ziglar.
Day 50	Make sure your goals are measurable, specific and time-bound. Having a measurable goal allows you to track your progress in smaller increments.
Day 51	Have a winner's mindset – it means you'll never give up.
Day 52	Remember there is a difference between weight loss and fat loss. Don't confuse this when jumping on the scales.
Day 53	When setting a fitness goal, focus on one objective at a time. Don't fall into the 'all or nothing' trap; slow and steady wins the race.
Day 54	Drink green tea to help increase your metabolism and burn more fat.
Day 55	Smiling more often, even when you don't feel like it, helps your body tackle and overcome stressful situations.

Day 56	Pumping iron isn't the only way to get lean muscle, give sprinting a go.
Day 57	Learn to let go. Tune into your mind and listen to what the universe is telling you.
Day 58	After periods of fasting, the hormone insulin becomes more effective in telling cells to take up glucose from the bloodstream for energy rather than for 'storage'.
Day 59	Sprints are a great way to burn fat, remember to slowly up the ante each time, to go from good to great.
Day 60	Make sure you're putting your mind in the muscle when it comes to training – feel the burn.
Day 62	A 24-hour fast is a great way to rethink your eating habits. By incorporating this ritual each week, your body will change.
Day 63	Fat loss means reducing your body-fat percentage – the amount of fat you carry. Weight loss means reducing your overall bodyweight. Aim for fat loss; don't get caught up in the numbers on the scale.
Day 64	Release the endorphins. When you smile, your brain releases tiny molecules called neuropeptides to help fight stress and creates a positive ripple effect.

Day 65	Enjoy increased flexibility, lower blood pressure and calmness with Hatha Yoga. Watch the bonus video at leanmuscle.com.
Day 66	Tailor that training outfit for both comfort and looks. It gets you in a focused mindset and you'd be surprised how much it helps to optimise your efforts.
Day 67	Sweet potatoes are a great source of fibre, vitamins and minerals.
Day 68	Exercise helps your cardiovascular system work more efficiently, which increases your energy levels for any activity.
Day 69	Grapefruit is a rich source of vitamin C and great for the immune system. It contains pectin, a form of soluble fibre that helps cholesterol.
Day 70	Include essential fatty acids (EFAs) in your diet; they have so many positive effects at a biological level.
Day 71	Workout as early as you can in the morning, often you're less prone to distractions, plus it's easier to do the hard stuff on your to-do list first up.
Day 72	Positive thinking copes with stress faster and more effectively than entertaining those pesky negative thoughts. Fight them off relentlessly.

Day 73	Next time you train, try taking shorter rest periods if you want to increase your calorie burn, or try lifting in a slightly lower rep range if you really want to build strength.
Day 74	Don't train to muscle failure: it only sets you up to fail.
Day 75	Forget 90% diet for fat loss; keep hacking your central nervous system with a combination of good sleep, good thoughts, good breath work and meditation, good nutrition knowledge and lots of daily movement and exercise.
Day 76	Eat your greens every day, you can't go wrong.
Day 77	Sweat Swear and Smile is the mantra for today.
Day 78	Another benefit to eating less food is a positive impact on the environment. The modern western world over-consumes; we need to better balance the land use between farming and environmental needs for the planet's ecosystems.
Day 79	Time to check in on that buddy again. Are they still keeping you accountable? Thank them for being on this journey with you.

Day 80	A positive mindset means that you have a positive expectation that things will turn out well and that you will succeed.
Day 81	You're on the home stretch – well-done – super proud of you!
Day 82	With certainty comes clarity. You have developed tools to take with you for the rest of your life.
Day 83	As your coach I couldn't be prouder! You are now on the road to even greater change and fulfillment.
Day 84	I hope these little tips have been timely reminders for you along your 12-Week Challenge. Take your final 'after' pictures and load them in the system. I commend you for taking the time to transform your life. It's onwards and upwards from here. Remember keep testing and measuring in your own life. Congratulations!

www.ingramcontent.com/pod-product-compliance
Lightning Source LLC
Chambersburg PA
CBHW071612080526
44588CB00010B/1101